HANDBOOK
OF CLINICAL
ELECTROCARDIOGRAPHY

HANDBOOK
OF CLINICAL
ELECTROCARDIOGRAPHY

Dr Tapas Kumar Koley MBBS, MD (Internal Medicine)
(Gold Medalist)
Formerly Senior Medical Officer, Hindu Rao Hospital, Delhi
Specialist Physician, Tilak Nagar Colony Hospital
Tilak Nagar, New Delhi

New Central Book Agency (P) Ltd
LONDON
DELHI KOLKATA PUNE HYDERABAD ERNAKULAM

REGD. OFFICE

8/1 Chintamoni Das Lane, Kolkata 700 009, India
email: ncbapvtltd@eth.net

OVERSEAS

27 Catherine Court, Chase Road, Southgate, London, N14 4RB

EXPORT

212 Shahpur Jat, New Delhi 110 049
email: ncbaexp@ncbapvtltd.com

BRANCHES

4262/3 1st Floor, Flat Nos. 105 & 106
Ansari Road, Daryaganj, New Delhi 110 002
email: ncbadel@ncbapvtltd.com

House No. 3-1-315, 1st Floor
Nimboliadda, Kachiguda, Hyderabad 500 027
email: ncbahydb@ncbapvtltd.com

Shop Nos. 3 & 4, Vinayak Towers
681/B Budhwar Peth, Appa Balwant Chowk
Pune 411 002
email: ncbapune@ncbapvtltd.com

GSS Shopping Complex, 1st Floor
Opposite College Post Office, Convent Road
Ernakulam 682 035
email: ncbaernk@ncbapvtltd.com

Handbook of Clinical Electrocardiography

First Published: July 2009

PUBLISHER

New Central Book Agency (P) Ltd
8/1 Chintamoni Das Lane, Kolkata 700 009

TYPESETTER

Tele Vijay Technologies (P) Ltd, Chennai

PRINTER

New Central Book Agency (P) Ltd
Web-Offset Division, Dhulagarh, Sankrail, Howrah

COVER DESIGNER
Soumen Paul

COVER PRINTER
Liba Graphics, Kolkata

ISBN: 978-81-7381-603-1

Price: [Three Hundred and Eighty-five]
56. 00

PREFACE

There are considerable developments in the field of electrocardio-gram (ECG). There are several voluminous textbooks on ECG with exhaustive details that often make the subject very confusing especially for the beginners. Keeping these facts in mind, this book is written to assist medical students, physicians, nurses, nursing students, paramedics, emergency medical technicians, and other allied health personnel in acquiring knowledge essential for identifying basic ECG abnormalities. Important features are marked in the ECG strips with arrows for easy understanding. Several colourful diagrams are provided to make the text easy to understand.

The book is conveniently divided into 11 chapters with a glossary at the end that covers all the important information about ECG. The language is very simple and lucid. The chapters emphasize the topics that have compelling practical application. All the important and related information is highlighted in the boxes, which I hope will help the readers to understand the subject better. The calculation of QRS axis has been described in the simplest possible manner, which I hope, will be of immense help to the beginners.

I have made every attempt to check the content of the book, for accuracy. I accept full responsibility for any error of omission or commission and welcome active criticism of the book.

7 May 2009   **Tapas Kumar Koley**
New Delhi, India

ACKNOWLEDGEMENT

A thanks giving although a pleasant job is also a difficult one when one sincerely tries to express them in words. These humble words, expressions, and gratitude cannot really convey the feelings of my heart. All the same, I am attempting to express my gratitude here.

At the very beginning, I am extremely grateful to my wife Mrs. Ruby Koley for providing me her constant support and encouragement while writing this book. She took a lot of burden on herself and made it easy for me to concentrate fully on the task of writing.

I am extremely thankful to Mr. R. K. Majumdar who has painstakingly drawn the diagrams for this book. Without his valuable help and priceless suggestions, it would not have been possible for me to complete this book.

I also express my sincere gratitude to my publisher "New Central Book Agency" for their sincere efforts in publishing and distributing this book. In preparation of this book, I have utilized the knowledge of a number of experts and consultants in my profession, and consulted many books and publications. I sincerely express my appreciation and gratitude to all of them.

Many others have contributed to and assisted in the perfection and completion of this work in various ways. I express my gratitude to all of them although they cannot be mentioned by their names here.

7 May 2009   **Tapas Kumar Koley**
New Delhi, India

LIST OF ABBREVIATIONS

APC	Atrial premature complex
ASD	Atrial septal defect
AV	Atrioventricular
BBB	Bundle branch block
CAH	Combined atrial hypertrophy
CVH	Combined ventricular hypertrophy
ECG	Electrocardiograph (UK)
EKG	Electrokardiograph (USA)
LA	Left atrium
LAD	Left axis deviation
LAH	Left atrial hypertrophy
LBBB	Left bundle branch block
LGL	Lown-Ganong-Levine
LV	Left ventricle
LVH	Left ventricular hypertrophy
PAT	Paroxysmal atrial tachycardia
PDA	Patent ductus arteriosus
PSVT	Paroxysmal supraventricular tachycardia
QTc	Corrected QT interval
RA	Right atrium
RAD	Right axis deviation
RAH	Right atrial hypertrophy
RBBB	Right bundle branch block
RV	Right ventricle
RVH	Right ventricular hypertrophy
SA	Sinoatrial
SSS	Sick sinus syndrome
SVT	Supraventricular tachycardia
VF	Ventricular fibrillation
VSD	Ventricular septal defect
VT	Ventricular tachycardia
WPW	Wolf-Parkinson-White

CONTENTS

CHAPTER 1

Basic Principles of Electrocardiography

Chapter Outline

INTRODUCTION

The invention of the electrocardiograph by Dutch physiologist Willem Einthoven in 1902 opened up a new way for the observation of cardiac electrical activity and a new chapter was written in the field of diagnosis of cardiac pathology. Since its invention, it has been used for diagnosis of various cardiac ailments.

An electrocardiogram (ECG) is the graphical recording of the change in potentials of the electrical field produced by the heart. ECG is used to study the cardiac anatomy and physiology. It helps in diagnosis of cardiac arrhythmias, conduction defects, myocardial hypertrophy, ischaemia, infarction, congenital heart diseases etc. It should be always kept in mind that ECG is only a laboratory test. A patient with heart disease may have a normal ECG and a normal healthy person may show non-specific changes in ECG. The ECG should be interpreted after examination of the patient and should be interpreted after analyzing the clinical findings.

ELECTROPHYSIOLOGY

The human heart is made up of four chambers: right atrium, left atrium, right ventricle and left ventricle. The two atria are separated by inter-atrial septum and the two ventricles are separated by interventricular septum (Fig. 1.1). The function of the heart is to pump blood to various organs of the body by contracting and relaxing in an orderly sequence.

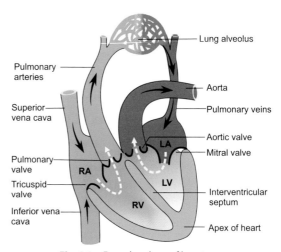

Fig. 1.1   Four chambers of heart.

There is a potential difference of approximately −90 mV across the cell membrane due to the presence of sodium–potassium pump. The outside of the cell is positively charged and the inside is negatively charged (as compared with each other) due to variable distribution of sodium and potassium ions (Fig. 1.2).

The cardiac muscle (e.g., sinoatrial node) has the property of automatic rhythmic contraction. Whenever an impulse is generated, the positive ions flow inside the cell and the region becomes positive as compared with outer region (which becomes negative), i.e., phase 0 of action potential. This process is called the depolarization of the cell (Fig. 1.3). During recovery, the positive ions are pumped out of the cell and again the inner region of the cell becomes negative as compared with the outer region (which becomes positive) and this process is called repolarization (Fig. 1.4). This depolarization is transmitted to the adjoining cells and a moving wavefront of depolarization is produced. This generates electric current, which is amplified and recorded as ECG.

After depolarization there is repolarization of the cardiac cell. At this stage, the cell is in a state where it can be further excited

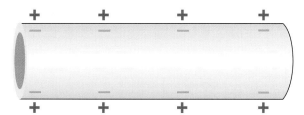

Fig. 1.2 Myocardial cell. At resting state, the outer region of the cell is positively charged and the inner region of the cell is negatively charged as compared with each other.

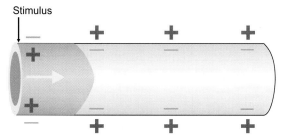

Fig. 1.3 Depolarization of cardiac cell. During depolarization, the inner region of the cell becomes positive and the outer region becomes negative due to rapid influx of sodium ions.

by a proper stimulus. Depolarization and repolarization occurs in both atrial and ventricular muscles and the whole process is very well synchronized that the atria and ventricles contract and relax in a rhythmic manner. However, depolarization and repolarization are electrical events and are not equal to systole and diastole. Depolarization just precedes systole and repolarization just precedes diastole.

An electrode facing the wave of depolarization records a positive (upright) deflection whereas an electrode from which the wave of depolarization is moving away records a negative (downward) deflection (Fig. 1.5). An impulse moving perpendicularly to an

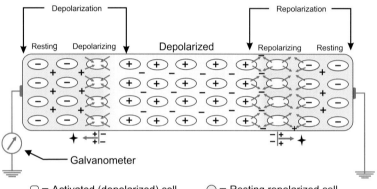

Fig. 1.4   The electrical events of depolarization and repolarization.

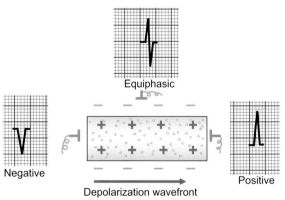

Fig. 1.5   Basic principle of generation of positive, negative, and equiphasic deflections. An impulse moving towards the electrode produces positive (upright) deflection and an impulse moving away from the electrode produces negative (downward) deflection.

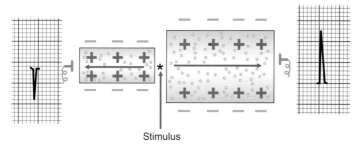

Stimulus

Fig. 1.6   Generation of waves in two muscle masses of markedly different size. A large positive deflection occurs towards the bigger muscle mass and a negative deflection occurs towards the smaller muscle mass.

electrode will produce a partly positive and a partly negative (biphasic/equiphasic) deflection.

If two muscle masses of markedly different sizes are stimulated at a central point, then a large positive wave will be recorded over the bigger muscle mass and a large negative deflection will result over the smaller muscle mass (Fig. 1.6).

ELECTROCARDIOGRAPH PAPER

ECG paper is in the form of a grid in which the horizontal and vertical lines are separated by 1 mm. Every fifth line in both the directions is darker than the other lines. The small squares are 1 mm^2 the large squares are 5 mm^2. The horizontal axis represents the time at 25 mm/s paper speed. One millimetre represents 0.04 s and five millimetre represents 0.2 s. The vertical axis represents the amplitude. At normal standardization (10 mm = 1 mV), each millimetre represents 0.1mV (Fig. 1.7). The ECG conventions are summarized in Box 1.1.

Box 1.1   Basic ECG Conventions
• Speed of paper: 25 mm/s
• Each small square: 0.04 s in horizontal axis
• Standardization: 10 mm = 1 mV
• Each small square: 0.1 mV in vertical axis
• Depolarization wavefront moving towards the electrode: Positive or upwards deflection
• Depolarization wavefront moving away from the electrode: Negative or downwards deflection

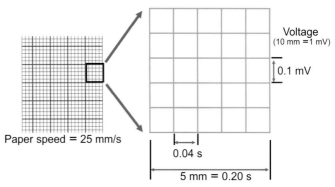

Fig. 1.7   Enlarged view of ECG paper showing time and voltage.

ELECTROCARDIOGRAPH LEADS

ECG leads are the pairs of electrodes across which the electrical potential is measured. There are 12 conventional leads which are divided into frontal plane and horizontal plane leads.

1. Frontal plane leads—Standard leads I, II, III, and leads aVR, aVL, and aVF.
2. Horizontal plane leads—Precordial leads V1–V6.

Frontal Plane Leads

Standard Leads

The electrodes are placed at the extremities, i.e., the right arm, the left arm, and the left leg. The electrical potential recorded from one extremity will be same irrespective of where the electrode is placed on the extremity. If the limbs are amputated, then the electrodes are placed on the amputated stumps. If the patient is suffering from tremor or shivering, then the electrodes should be placed at the upper end of the limbs.

1. Standard lead I—Produced by placing the positive electrode on left arm and the negative electrode on the right arm.
2. Standard lead II—Produced by placing the positive electrode on the left foot and the negative electrode on the right arm.
3. Standard lead III—Produced by placing the positive electrode on left foot and negative electrode on the left arm.

It may be noted that the left foot is always positive and the right arm is always negative as far as the placement of electrodes is concerned. Standard lead II is commonly used for cardiac monitoring as positioning of electrodes most commonly resembles the pathway of current flow in normal atrial and ventricular depolarization.

An imaginary line joining the positive and negative electrodes of a lead is called the axis of the lead. The three lead axes of these three leads form an equilateral triangle with the heart at centre called Einthoven's triangle (Fig. 1.8).

Unipolar Augmented Limb Leads

According to Einthoven's law, the sum of the potentials of the three lead axes is equal to zero. When these three leads are connected the potential of that terminal is zero. This is the central terminal (indifferent electrode). When this terminal is connected to one pole of the galvanometer, the potential at that pole will be zero. The electrode (exploring electrode) attached to the other pole of galvanometer will record the potential at any point relative to the indifferent electrode. The voltage at the exploring electrode is augmented by disconnecting the indifferent electrode from the limb which is tested.

1. aVR—Right arm
2. aVL—Left arm
3. aVF—Left foot

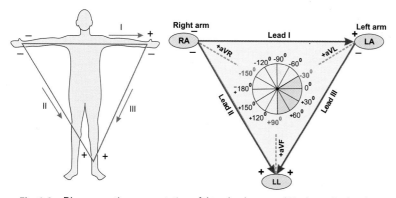

Fig. 1.8   Diagrammatic representation of three lead axes and Einthoven's triangle.

The 'a' stands for augmentation, i.e., the voltage is augmented by 50%.

Horizontal Plane Leads

The chest leads are represented by the letter 'V'. The placement is as follows (Fig. 1.9):

1. V1—Placed at the 4th intercostal space immediately to the right of sternum.
2. V2—Placed at the 4th intercostal space immediately to the left of sternum.
3. V3—Placed between leads V2 and V4.
4. V4—Placed at the 5th intercostal space on the left midclavicular line.
5. V5—Placed at the same horizontal level as that of lead V4 on the left anterior axillary line.
6. V6—Placed at the same horizontal level as that of leads V4 and V5 on the left midaxillary line.

The placement of leads is summarized in Box 1.2.

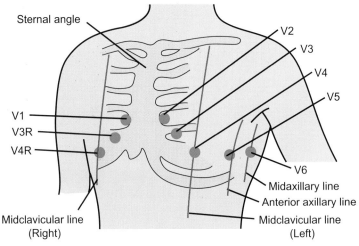

Fig. 1.9   Diagram showing the position of chest leads.

Box 1.2 Lead Placement

- Lead I: Left arm positive, right arm negative
- Lead II: Left foot positive, right arm negative
- Lead III: Left foot positive, left arm negative
- aVR: Right arm
- aVL: Left arm
- aVF: Left foot
- V1: Right 4th intercostal space by the side of sternum
- V2: Left 4th intercostal space by the side of sternum
- V3: Between leads V2 and V4
- V4: Left 5th intercostal space on midclavicular line
- V5: Same horizontal plane as lead V4 on anterior axillary line
- V6: Same horizontal plane as lead V4 and V5 on midaxillary line
- V7: Same horizontal plane as lead V4 on posterior axillary line
- V8: Same horizontal plane as lead V4 on posterior scapular line
- V9: Same horizontal plane as lead V4 on posterior left border of spine
- V3R–V9R: Same position as leads V3–V9 but on right side of chest

RECORDING OF ECG

1. Patient must lie down comfortably and relax. Tell him/her the procedure and you must explain that he will not feel any electric current.
2. Wipe the patient's skin with alcohol and allow it to dry. Then apply the conductive gel and connect the proper electrodes and ensure that they are in good contact with the skin.
3. The patient and the machine must be properly grounded. Any electronic equipment may produce artefacts and hence should be removed.
4. Calibrate the record (1 mV = 10 mm).
5. Record the six standard leads.
6. Record the six chest leads.

STANDARDIZATION OF ECG

Standardization of ECG is one of the most important and over-looked aspect of ECG. Before analysing an ECG it is most important to look for proper standardization. If the standardization is

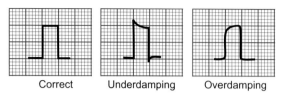

| Correct | Underdamping | Overdamping |

Fig. 1.10   Diagram showing normal standardization, overdamping, and overshoot.

not correct, then there is a possibility of wrong diagnosis of right ventricular hypertrophy or left ventricular hypertrophy (due to increase in the amplitude of R or S waves) or old myocardial infarction (due to increase in the amplitude of physiological q waves) or pericardial effusion (due to low amplitude of R and S waves).

Conventionally, ECG is standardized so that 1 mV is equal to 10 mm of upward deflection.

Overdamping—It occurs when the stylus presses too much on the paper (and platform) resulting in rounded corners. It leads to widening of the complex.

Underdamping or overshoot—It occurs when the stylus is too loose resulting in spikes at the corners. It results in increase in amplitude of the complex (see Fig. 1.10).

BIBLIOGRAPHY

1. Braunwald E. (ed). *Heart Disease: A Textbook of Cardiovascular Medicine*, Fifth edition, W.B. Saunders Co.: Philadelphia, PA, 1997; pp. 119–123.
2. Burger HC and Van Milaan JB. Heart-vector and leads. *Br Heart J* 1946; 8, 157–161.
3. Fye WB. A history of the origin, evolution, and impact of electrocardiography. *Am J Cardiol* 1994; 73, 937–949.
4. Goldberger E. *Unipolar Lead Electrocardiography*, Second edition, Lea & Febiger: Philadelphia, PA, 1950.
5. Helm RA and Chou TC. Electrocardiographic leads. *Am J Cardiol* 1964; 14, 317–329.
6. Rudy Y. The ionic mechanisms of conduction in cardiac tissue. *J Electrocardiol* 2001; 34(suppl), 65–68.
7. Schamroth L. *An Introduction to Electrocardiography*, Seventh edition, Blackwell Science (Indian Reprint), UK, 2002; pp. 5–33.

CHAPTER 2

Normal Electrocardiogram

NOMENCLATURE OF ELECTROCARDIOGRAM WAVES

The nomenclature of the electrocardiogram (ECG) waves is arranged alphabetically as P, Q, R, S, T, and U (Fig. 2.1). The capital letters represent big waves (more than 5 mm) and the small letters represent smaller waves (less than 5 mm).

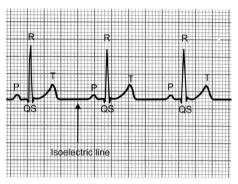

Fig. 2.1 Nomenclature of waves of an ECG.

WAVES AND COMPLEXES

Normal Components of an ECG Complex
The normal components of an ECG complex are

1. Waveforms: P, QRS, T, U waves
2. Intervals: P–R, R–R, Q–T, P–P intervals, and QRS duration
3. Junction: QRS–T junction called J point
4. Segments: S–T segment

P Wave
P wave is produced by depolarization of both the right and the left atria. It is the first wave of the ECG (Fig. 2.2). The first part of P wave reflects the depolarization of the right atrium and the second part reflects the depolarization of the left atrium. It is smooth and rounded and best seen in lead II. The duration is 0.08–0.10 s. The maximum amplitude and duration is 2.5 mm. The P wave may be biphasic, flat, or inverted in lead V1.

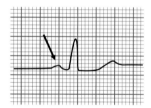

Fig. 2.2 P wave (arrow).

Ta or Pt Wave
Ta or Pt wave is due to atrial repolarization and is usually not visible (Fig. 2.3).

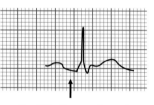

Fig. 2.3 Ta wave (arrow).

QRS Complex

QRS complex is the major ECG deflection and is produced by synchronous depolarization of both the ventricles. The QRS complex is positive in all leads but lead aVR. A normal QRS complex has smooth limbs with no notch or slurring (Fig. 2.4).

Q Wave

The first negative deflection after P wave is known as Q wave (Fig. 2.5a, b). It precedes the first positive deflection (R wave) of the QRS complex. It is produced by depolarization of the ventricular septum from left to right. A normal Q wave has duration of less than 0.04 s, less than 25% of the height of R wave in the same complex and

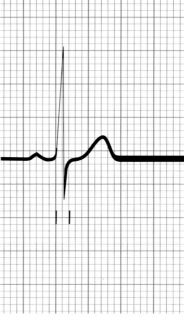

Fig. 2.4 Normal QRS complex. Duration: 0.08 s (2 squares × 0.04 s).

is less than 4 mm deep. It is normally visible in leads I, aVL, V5, and V6. The normal Q wave is represented by 'q' and may not be seen in all the leads.

R Wave

R wave is the first positive deflection of the QRS complex (Fig. 2.6). Usually, in the limb leads, the height of R wave is at least 5 mm and in the chest leads the height of R wave is at least 10 mm. In lead

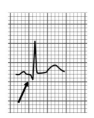

Fig. 2.5a q wave (arrow).

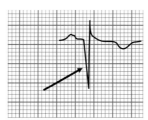

Fig. 2.5b Q wave (arrow).

V1, the height of R wave is less and gradually the height increases from lead V1 to V6. This is called progression of the R wave amplitude.

S Wave

S wave is the first negative deflection of the QRS complex after R wave. It is the terminal part of ventricular depolarization (Fig. 2.7). The magnitude of S wave in lead V1 is more than the height of R wave and in lead V6 the magnitude of S wave is much less than the height of R wave.

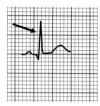

Fig. 2.6   R wave (arrow).

R' Wave

R´ wave is the second positive deflection after the R wave (Fig. 2.8). It is seen during bundle branch block.

S' Wave

S´ wave is the second negative deflection after the S wave (Fig. 2.9). It is also seen during bundle branch block.

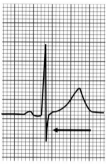

Fig. 2.7   S wave (arrow).

T Wave

T wave is seen after the QRS complex and is produced by ventricular repolarization. It has asymmetric limbs with a blunt apex and is in the same direction as that of the QRS complex (Fig. 2.10). It is normally upright in all the leads with exception of aVR where it

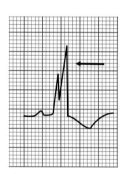

Fig. 2.8   R' wave (arrow).

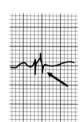

Fig. 2.9   S' wave (arrow).

Fig. 2.10   T wave (arrow).

is inverted. It is often inverted in lead V1. The normal T wave does not exceed 5 mm in limb leads and 10 mm in chest leads.

U Wave

The genesis of U wave is uncertain and probably represents the slow repolarization of the Purkinje fibres. It occurs after the T wave and is in the same direction as that of the T wave but much less in amplitude (Fig. 2.11). It is best seen in leads V2–V4. U wave more than 2 mm is considered abnormal and may be due to hypokalaemia or digitalis effect.

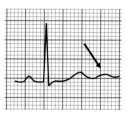

Fig. 2.11   U wave (arrow).

TIME INTERVALS

Various time intervals and segments are studied while reading an ECG. The important ones are the following:

1. P–R interval
2. P–R segment
3. P–P interval
4. R–R interval
5. QRS interval
6. S–T segment
7. Q–T interval

P–R Interval

It is the time interval between the beginning of P wave and beginning of Q wave or R wave (in the absence of Q wave) of the QRS complex (Fig. 2.12a). The QRS complex may begin with either R wave or q wave. If there is a q wave, then it is measured from the beginning of P wave to the beginning of q wave of the qRS complex. It denotes the time interval between atrial depolarization and ventricular depolarization. It is mainly contributed by atrioventricular (AV) nodal delay in conduction of the impulse.

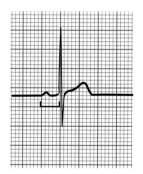

Fig. 2.12a   P–R interval. In this electrocardiogram (ECG), the P–R interval is 5 × 0.04 s = 0.20 s.

It includes the time for:

1. Atrial depolarization.
2. Normal conduction delay of the AV node (0.07 s).
3. The passage of impulse through bundle of His and bundle branches to the onset of ventricular depolarization.

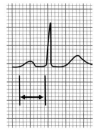

Normal P–R interval is 0.12–0.2 s. However, the P–R interval must be correlated with the heart rate, the slower the heart rate the longer is the P–R interval. Prolonged P–R interval (Fig. 2.12b) is seen in first-degree heart block and shortened P–R interval is seen in Wolf–Parkinson–White syndrome and Lown–Ganong–Levine syndrome.

Fig. 2.12b P–R interval. In this ECG, the P–R interval is 7 × 0.04 s = 0.28 s.

P–R Segment

P–R segment is part of the P–R interval. It is that part of the isoelectric line that starts from the end of the P wave to the beginning of the QRS complex. It does not include the P wave (Fig. 2.13). It allows time for the atria to empty blood into the ventricles before ventricular contraction begins.

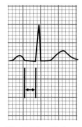

Fig. 2.13 P–R segment.

P–P Interval

P–P interval is the time interval between two successive P waves. It is calculated from the beginning of one P wave to the beginning of the next P wave. It helps in calculating atrial rate. In normal sinus rhythm, this interval is equal to the R–R interval.

R–R Interval

R–R interval is the time interval between two successive R waves (Fig. 2.14). It helps in calculating ventricular rate (heart rate). A slight variation in the R–R interval, due to the effect of respiration, is usually considered normal.

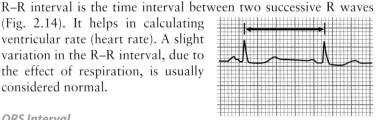

Fig. 2.14 R–R interval. In this electrocardiogram, the R–R interval is 22 × 0.04 s = 0.88 s.

QRS Interval

QRS interval is also called QRS duration. It is measured from the beginning

Box 2.1   Causes of Wide QRS Complex

- Bundle branch block
- Intraventricular conduction delay
- Wolf–Parkinson–White syndrome
- Ventricular premature beat
- Idioventricular rhythm
- Ventricular tachycardia.

of Q wave to the end of S wave or 'j' point (junction of S wave and S–T segment). It represents the total time taken for ventricular depolarization (Fig. 2.15). In the absence of Q wave, the interval is measured from the origin of the R wave. The normal upper limit is 0.1 s and is prolonged in various conditions (Box 2.1).

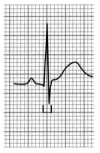

Fig. 2.15 QRS interval. In this electrocardiogram, the QRS duration is 0.04 s × 2 = 0.08 s.

S–T Segment

S–T segment starts at the 'j' (junction) point and ends at the beginning of T wave (Figs. 2.16 and 2.17). It represents ventricular repolarization. S–T segment is isoelectric and represents phase 2 of repolarization, i.e., plateau phase. One millimetre S–T segment elevation is normal in leads I, II, and III and up to two millimetre elevation is normal in some precordial leads (in the absence of symptoms of myocardial infarction). S–T segment elevation in only one lead is not diagnostic of any disease.

Q–T Interval

Q–T interval is measured from the beginning of Q wave to the end of T wave (Figs. 2.18 and 2.19). In the absence of Q wave, the

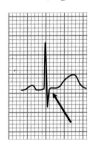
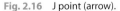

Fig. 2.16   J point (arrow).

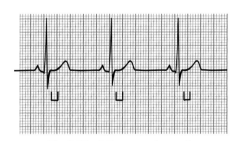

Fig. 2.17   S–T segment (normal).

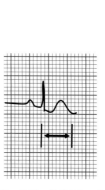

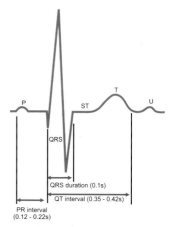

Fig. 2.18   Q–T interval. In this ECG, the Q–T interval is 0.04 s × 8 = 0.32 s.

Fig. 2.19   A normal QRS complex with nomenclature and various time intervals.

interval is measured from the beginning of R wave to the end of T wave. It represents the duration of ventricular systole, i.e., depolarization plus repolarization. Q–T interval varies with heart rate. It increases during bradycardia and shortens during tachycardia. Q–T interval corrected for heart rate is called Q–T$_c$.

$$Q\text{–}T_c = \frac{Q\text{–}T}{\sqrt{R\text{–}R} \ \text{interval}} \qquad \text{(Bazett's formula)}$$

The value of Q–T$_c$ corresponds to the Q–T interval at a heart rate of 60 beats/min. The normal range of Q–T$_c$ is 0.35–0.42 s. It is longer in females and in old age. Prolonged Q–T interval may lead to a special type of ventricular tachycardia called Torsades de Pointes.

POINTS TO REMEMBER

1.   At a heart rate of 60 beats/min, Q–T is the same as Q–T$_c$.
2.   At a heart rate of 60–100 beats/min, Q–T interval should not be more than half of the R–R interval.

The various causes of abnormal Q–T$_c$ are summarized in Box 2.2 and the various time intervals are summarized in Box 2.3.

Ventricular Activation Time
Ventricular activation time (VAT) is the time taken by an impulse to travel from endocardium to epicardium. It is measured from

Box 2.2   Abnormal Q–T$_c$

Prolonged Q–T$_c$
- Hypocalcaemia
- Quinidine and procainamide effects
- Acute myocardial infarction
- Acute myocarditis
- Deep sleep
- Hypothermia
- Torsades de Pointes
- Tricyclic antidepressant drugs
- Congenital—prolonged Q–T syndrome, Romano–Ward syndrome
- Electrolyte imbalance
  (a) Hypokalaemia
  (b) Hypomagnesaemia
- CVA (Cerebrovascular accident)
- Idiopathic

Shortened Q–T$_c$
- Digitalis effect
- Hypercalcaemia
- Hyperthermia
- Phenytoin sodium therapy

Box 2.3   Various Time Intervals

- QRS interval: 0.1 s
- P–R interval: 0.12–0.2 s
- Ventricular activation time: 0.02 s in lead VI to 0.05 s in lead V6
- Q–T$_c$: 0.35 s to 0.42 s
- Heart rate: 1,500/R–R interval

the beginning of Q wave to the peak of the R wave (Fig. 2.20). Normally it is 0.02 s in lead V1 and 0.04–0.05 s in lead V6. VAT increases in ventricular hypertrophy.

CALCULATION OF HEART RATE

Calculation of heart rate in ECG implies ventricular rate. This in turn means number of QRS complexes per minute. The atrial rate

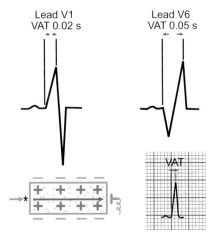

Fig. 2.20   Ventricular activation time (VAT).

can be calculated from the P–P interval and the ventricular rate can be calculated from the R–R interval. In sinus rhythm, both are same but during arrhythmia they have to be calculated separately.

Regular Rhythm

When the rhythm is regular, the heart rate may be calculated by calculating the R–R interval.

Heart rate = 1,500/R–R interval. This is true when the paper speed is at 25 mm/s. [For example, if the R–R interval is 10 (10 smallest squares) then heart rate = 1,500/10 = 150 beats/min.].

If the R–R interval is such that the peak of R wave coincides with the dark vertical lines of ECG paper, then just count the number of bigger squares (5 mm squares) in the R–R interval and then divide 300 with the number of bigger squares. This is true when the rhythm is regular and the paper speed is 25 mm/s (Fig. 2.21). (For example, if the number of bigger squares in the R–R interval is 3, then the heart rate is 300/3 = 100 beats/min.).

Irregular Rhythm

When rhythm is irregular, then rapid rate calculation is done by 6-second method. In this method, count the number of R waves in a 6-second strip (i.e., thirty 5 mm squares) and then multiply it by 10. This will give the heart rate per minute (Fig. 2.22).

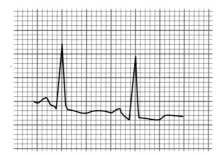

Fig. 2.21   Calculation of heart rate. The number of small squares in between the two 'R' waves is 15. Therefore, the heart rate (ventricular rate) is 1,500/15 = 100 beats/min. In the other method, the calculation will be 300/3 = 100 beats/min because there are three big squares between the two 'R' waves.

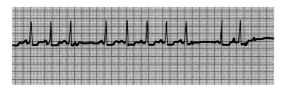

Fig. 2.22   Six-second method. In this strip, the number of R waves in 6 second (i.e., thirty 5 mm squares) is 10. Then heart rate is 10 × 10 = 100 beats/min.

GENESIS OF THE QRS COMPLEX

The first part of the ventricle to be activated is the interventricular septum. The activation starts at the subendocardial region of septum with the activation force spreading from left to right. This is the septal vector. This leads to small positive wave (r wave) in lead V1, i.e., the lead facing the wavefront and a small negative wave (q wave) in lead V6, i.e., the lead from which the wavefront is receding (Fig. 2.23).

After activation of the septum there is activation of free walls of both the ventricles. This occur transversely from endocardium to epicardium resulting in a large right to left wavefront (vector) because of thicker left ventricular myocardium and a small wavefront from left to right because of thinner right ventricular myocardium. These two vectors are opposite to each other and the larger vector neutralizes the smaller vector and, therefore, the resultant vector is directed from right to left. This leads to a deep negative wave in lead V1 (S wave) as the wavefront is receding away from this electrode and a large positive wave in lead V6 (R wave) as the wavefront is going towards the electrode (Fig. 2.24).

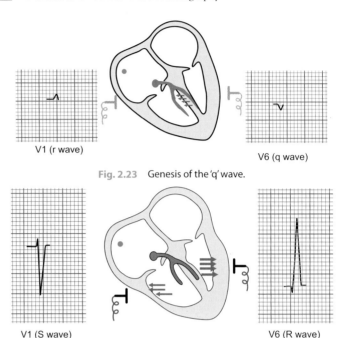

V1 (r wave)

V6 (q wave)

Fig. 2.23   Genesis of the 'q' wave.

V1 (S wave)

V6 (R wave)

Fig. 2.24   Genesis of R and S waves.

The transition zone is that area which records the transition from rS (in lead V1) to qR (in lead V6) pattern. It is usually lead V3 or V4 where the R and S waves are of same height and depth, respectively. It is to be remembered that in lead aVR all the waves are negative as the lead is directed to the cavity of the heart (Fig. 2.25). The geneses of the waves are summarized in Box 2.4.

ROTATION OF THE HEART

Rotation of the heart refers to rotation of the electrical forces and not the anatomical rotation. The heart rotates theoretically along two axes, the anteroposterior axis and the longitudinal axis. Rotation around the anteroposterior axis reflects the rotation along the frontal plane and rotation around the longitudinal axis reflects rotation in the horizontal plane.

Rotation Around the Anteroposterior Axis
The anteroposterior axis runs through the interventricular septum from the anterior to the posterior surface of the heart. The rotation

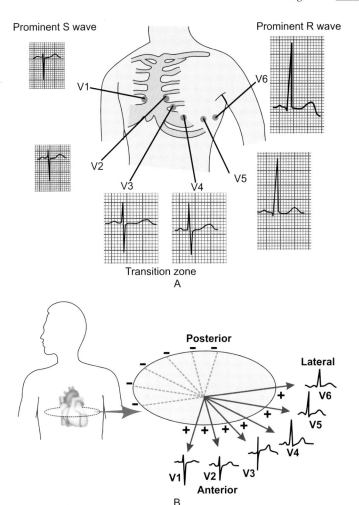

Fig. 2.25 ECG configuration in chest leads. (A) ECG complexes on an ECG paper. (B) Diagrammatic representation of ECG complexes in chest leads.

Box 2.4   Genesis of Waves

- P wave: Atrial depolarization
- Ta wave: Atrial repolarization
- QRS complex: Ventricular depolarization
- T wave: Ventricular repolarization
- U wave: Uncertain

of electrical forces of heart across an anteroposterior axis leads to three different positions of heart.

1. Vertical position
2. Horizontal position
3. Intermediate position

Vertical Position

Vertical position of heart is seen in tall and thin persons. The left ventricular complex is recorded in lead aVF. Therefore, PQRS complex of lead aVF resembles that of lead V6 (Fig. 2.26a, b). The mean QRS axis is directed inferiorly (=+75°).

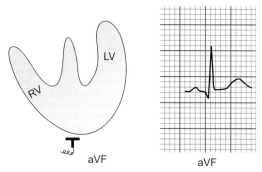

Fig. 2.26a   Diagram of vertical heart. LV, left ventricle; RV, right ventricle.

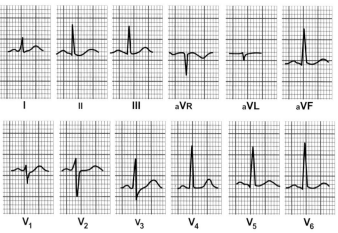

Fig. 2.26b   ECG showing vertical position of the heart. The QRS complex of aVF resembles that of V6.

Horizontal Position

Horizontal position of heart is seen in obese persons with broad chests. The left ventricular complex is recorded in lead aVL. The QRS complex in lead aVL resembles that of lead V6 (Fig. 2.27a, b). The mean QRS axis is between 0° and −30°.

Intermediate Position

Intermediate position of heart is midway between the vertical and horizontal position; both lead aVL and lead aVF resembles that of lead V6 (Fig. 2.28).

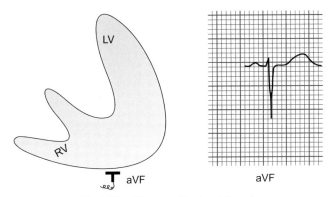

Fig. 2.27a   Diagram of horizontal heart.

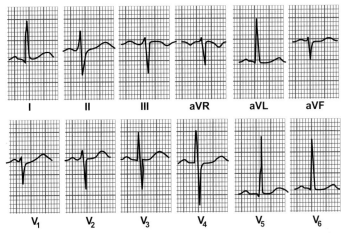

Fig. 2.27b   ECG showing horizontal position of the heart. The PQRS complex of lead aVL resembles that of lead V6.

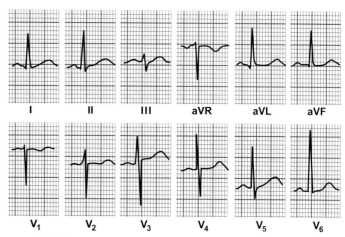

Fig. 2.28   ECG showing intermediate position of heart. The PQRS complex of both lead aVL and lead aVF resembles that of lead V6.

Rotation Around the Longitudinal Axis

The longitudinal axis runs through the interventricular septum from the apex to the base. Rotation is conventionally viewed from below the heart (through the diaphragm) looking upwards. Rotation around this axis leads to clockwise and counter clockwise rotations (Fig. 2.29).

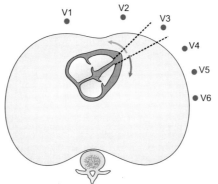

Fig. 2.29   Diagram showing rotation of the heart. Rotation along blue arrow leads to counter clockwise rotation and rotation along red arrow leads to clockwise rotation. Look at the heart from the foot end.

Clockwise Rotation

In clockwise rotation, the right ventricle is thought to come anteriorly and the interventricular septum becomes parallel to the chest wall. This means most of the chest leads will record an rS or RS complex and the transition zone will shift to lead V5 or V6 (Fig. 2.30). However, no such anatomical change occurs and it is merely the deviation of the electrical forces.

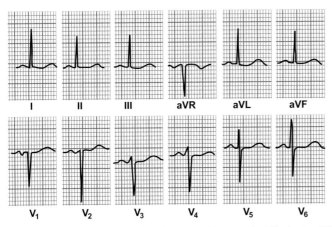

Fig. 2.30   ECG of clockwise rotation of the heart. Transition zone is shifted to lead V5.

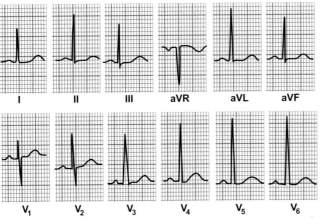

Fig. 2.31   ECG showing counter clockwise rotation of the heart. Transition zone is shifted to lead V1.

Counter Clockwise Rotation

Counter clockwise rotation brings the left ventricle more anteriorly. Here the changes will be opposite to that described in clockwise rotation and thus the transition zone is shifted to lead V1 or V2 (Fig. 2.31).

A normal ECG is shown in Fig. 2.32. The P, QRS and T waves in all the twelve leads are normal. All the waves are inverted in lead aVR. Transition zone is recorded in lead V3. The QRS axis is normal. The different time intervals are also within normal limit.

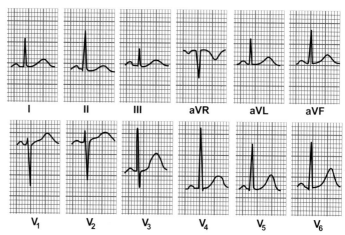

Fig. 2.32   Normal ECG. The QRS axis is normal. The rS complex is recorded in lead V1 and the qR complex is recorded in lead V6. Lead aVR reflects completely negative complex. Transition zone is recorded in lead V3.

In infants, the ECG will simulate that of right ventricular hypertrophy in adults. Tall R waves are present in the right precordial leads. There is right axis deviation. There is no initial q wave in lead V1 and the VAT is not prolonged. The T waves are normally inverted in leads V1–V4. The tall R waves in right precordial leads usually disappear after the age of 5, but the inverted T waves may persist even up to the second decade. The QRS axis gradually shifts to the left.

Artefacts are often observed in ECG. These are produced by sources other than the heart's electrical activity. The common causes are muscle tremor, shivering, loose electrodes, electrical equipment interference, improper grounding of ECG machine etc. (Fig. 2.33).

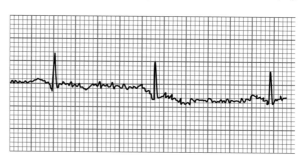

Fig. 2.33   ECG showing shivering artefacts. Note the irregular baseline. This ECG was taken from a patient of hypothermia due to exposure to cold water during winter.

BIBLIOGRAPHY

1. Bazett HC. An analysis of the time relations of electrocardio-grams. *Heart* 1920; 7, 353–370.
2. Cokkinos DV, Leachman RD, Zamalloa O, et al. Influence of atrial mass on amplitude and duration of the P wave. *Chest* 1972; 61, 336–339.
3. Leatham A. The chest lead electrocardiogram in health. *Br Heart J* 1950; 12, 213–231.
4. Schamroth L. *An Introduction to Electrocardiography*, Seventh edition, Blackwell Science (Indian Reprint), UK, 2002, pp. 121–128.
5. Scher AM. The sequence of ventricular excitation. *Am J Cardiol* 1964; 14, 287–293.
6. Steve M and Francis M. ABC of clinical electrocardiography. Introduction II—basic terminology. *BMJ* 2002; 324, 470–473.

CHAPTER 3

Electrical Axis

Chapter Outline

INTRODUCTION

Electrical axis means the direction of the net electrical force of the heart. In conditions such as left anterior hemiblock, left ventricular hypertrophy, Wolff–Parkinson–White syndrome, the axis calculation is extremely helpful in making a correct interpretation of the electrocardiogram (ECG).

The activation of the ventricles starts at the upper part of the interventricular septum. There is a small initial electrical wavefront (vector) from left to right. After that the free walls of the ventricles are activated and numerous vectors of various magnitude and direction are generated. *The vectors which are opposite to each other and of equal magnitude cancel each other.* The larger vectors dominate and the largest electrical force occurs near the apex of left ventricle and the adjoining left ventricular wall because of maximum muscle mass. It is mainly directed to the left and downwards. The dominant direction of all these multiple vectors is known as the mean vector and is expressed in ECG as the mean QRS axis.

AXIAL REFERENCE SYSTEM

Triaxial Reference System

The lead axes of the three standard limb leads are oriented in such a way that they form an equilateral triangle with the heart at its centre. This is known as Einthoven's triangle. If the lead axes are redrawn as shown in Fig. 3.1a (the three axes are passing through a common point), then these three lead axes form a triaxial reference system with each axis separated from the other by 60°. Note that the polarity and the orientation of the lead axes are not changed.

Similarly, another triaxial reference system is formed by the three lead axes of the augmented unipolar leads (Fig. 3.1b).

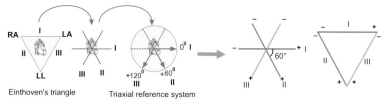

Einthoven's triangle   Triaxial reference system

Fig. 3.1a Diagram showing triaxial reference system formed by axis of limb leads.

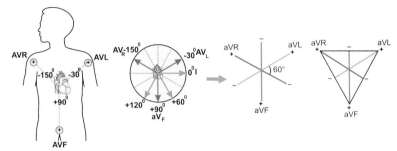

Fig 3.1b Diagram showing triaxial reference system formed by axis of augmented limb leads.

Hexaxial Reference System

When the two triaxial reference systems are combined and superimposed on each other, the hexaxial reference system is formed and the lead axes are separated from each other by 30° (Fig. 3.2). In this reference system, all the lead axes maintain their polarity and direction. By convention, the degrees in the upper half are labelled negative degrees (0° to –180°) and all the degrees in the lower half are labelled as positive (0° to +180°).

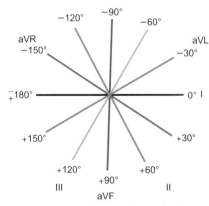

Fig. 3.2 Diagram showing hexaxial reference system formed by combination of two triaxial reference systems.

CALCULATION OF QRS AXIS

There is no unanimous agreement on the normal QRS axis. Some authors have mentioned it to be between –30° and +110° while others have calculated it to be between 0° and + 90°. The normal QRS axis lies between –30° and +90° (Meek S and Morris F., 2002). This data is used in this book. However, in most of the cases, the normal axis lies between +40° and +60°. For calculation of QRS axis, the hexaxial reference system is used. There are several methods mentioned in various ECG books. Many of them are quite confusing for the beginners. Here, only two simple methods will be described.

Method 1

If we consider Fig. 3.2, it may be noted that the lead axis of lead I and lead aVF is perpendicular to each other. The following steps are to be followed to calculate the QRS axis of the ECG (lead I and lead aVF are shown in Fig. 3.3).

Step I

Plot the lead axis of lead I and lead aVF.

Step II

Calculate the total positive and total negative deflection of the QRS complex in lead I. For example, it is +7 (R wave) and –2 (S wave) in the given ECG. So, the net deflection is +5 [+7+ (–2) = +5].

Now, plot +5 in the lead axis of lead I as shown in Fig. 3.4.

Step III

Draw a perpendicular through the plotted point on lead I axis as shown in Fig. 3.5.

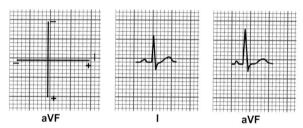

Fig. 3.3   Lead axis of lead I and lead aVF.

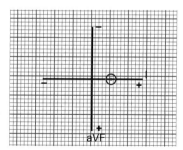

Fig. 3.4   Plotting of +5 on the axis of lead I.

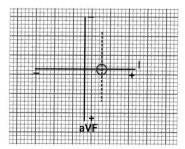

Fig. 3.5   Perpendicular drawn on lead I axis through +5.

Step IV

Now calculate the net deflection in lead aVF in the same method as described above. In the given ECG, the net deflection is +7 [+9+ (−2) = +7]. Now, plot +7 in the lead axis of lead aVF as shown in Fig. 3.6.

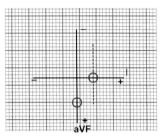

Fig. 3.6   Plotting of +7 on the axis of lead aVF.

Step V

Draw a perpendicular through the plotted point on lead aVF axis and prolong it to meet the perpendicular drawn on lead I axis as shown in Fig. 3.7.

Step VI

Draw a line joining the point of the intersection of the axis of lead I and lead aVF and the point of intersection of the two perpendicular lines. The QRS axis is +55° as shown in Fig. 3.8.

Method 2

This is a rapid method but gives only a rough estimation of the QRS axis. This is for those who already have a very clear concept of QRS axis and interpretation of ECG. Here also we have to look into the dominant QRS deflections in lead I and lead aVF. After this the interpretation is as follows:

Lead I	Lead aVF	QRS axis
Positive (R wave)	Positive (R wave)	Normal (−30° to +90°)
Positive (R wave)	Negative (S wave)	Left axis (−30° to −90°)
Negative (S wave)	Positive (R wave)	Right axis (+90° to +180°)
Negative (S wave)	Negative (S wave)	Northwest axis (−90° to −180°)

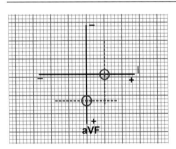

Fig. 3.7 Perpendicular drawn on axis of lead aVF through +7.

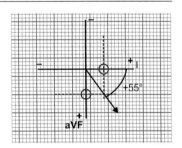

Fig. 3.8 QRS axis is +55°.

RIGHT AXIS DEVIATION

The normal QRS axis lies between −30° and +90° (Fig. 3.9). In right axis deviation, the QRS axis lies between +90° and +180° (+110° to +180° according to some other text books). It is seen in conditions like right bundle branch block, left posterior hemiblock, right ventricular hypertrophy. In left axis deviation, the axis is between −30° and −90°. Axis in northwest region is very rare.

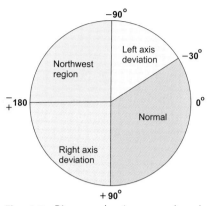

Fig. 3.9 Diagram showing normal and abnormal QRS axis.

Let us consider the QRS tracing in leads I and aVF of Fig. 3.10. There is a positive deflection in lead aVF and a negative deflection in lead I. If we calculate the QRS axis by the second method, then we can say that there is a deviation along the right axis but the exact axis can be determined only by the first method as described earlier. Let us calculate the axis by the first method and follow the steps as mentioned earlier.

Step I
Plot the lead axis of lead I and lead aVF.

Step II
Calculate the total positive and total negative deflection of the QRS complex in lead I. For example, it is +2 (r wave) and −14 (S wave) in the given ECG. So, the net deflection is −12 [+2+ (−14) = −12].

Now plot −12 in the lead axis of lead I as shown in Fig. 3.11.

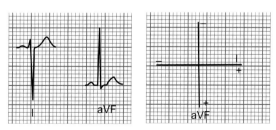

Fig. 3.10   Lead axis of lead I and lead aVF.

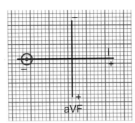

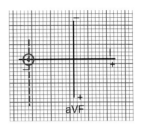

Fig. 3.11 Plotting of –12 on the axis of lead I.

Fig. 3.12 Perpendicular drawn on lead I axis through –12.

Step III

Draw a perpendicular through the plotted point on lead I axis as shown in Fig. 3.12.

Step IV

Now calculate the net deflection in lead aVF in the same manner. In the given ECG, the net deflection is +14 [+15+ (–1) = +14]. Now, plot +14 in the lead axis of lead aVF as shown in Fig. 3.13.

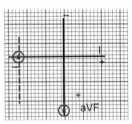

Fig. 3.13 Plotting of +14 on the axis of lead aVF.

Step V

Draw a perpendicular through the plotted point on lead aVF axis and prolong it to meet the perpendicular drawn on lead I axis as shown in Fig. 3.14.

Step VI

Draw a line joining the point of the inter-section of axis of lead I and lead aVF and

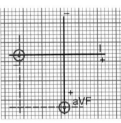

Fig. 3.14 Perpendicular drawn on axis of lead aVF through +14.

the point of intersection of the two perpendicular lines. The QRS axis is +132° as shown in Fig. 3.15.

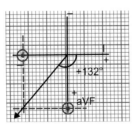

Fig. 3.15 The exact calculated axis is +132° (right axis deviation).

LEFT AXIS DEVIATION

Left axis deviation occurs when the QRS axis lies between –30° and –90°. QRS axis between –90° and –180° is very rare. Here also let us consider the QRS tracing of

Fig. 3.16. At a glance, using the second method we can say that there is left axis deviation but to calculate the exact axis, the first method has to be followed.

Step I
Plot the lead axis of lead I and lead aVF (Fig. 3.16).

Step II
Calculate the total positive and total negative deflection of the QRS complex in lead I. For example, it is +12 (R wave) and –2 (s wave) in the given ECG. So, the net deflection is +10 [+12+ (–2) = +10].

Now plot +10 in the lead axis of lead I as shown in the Fig. 3.17.

Step III
Draw a perpendicular through the plotted point on lead I axis as shown in Fig. 3.18.

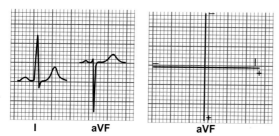

Fig. 3.16   Lead axis of lead I and lead aVF.

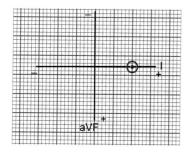

Fig. 3.17   Plotting of +10 on the axis of lead I.

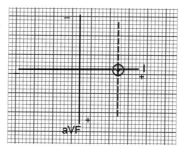

Fig. 3.18   Perpendicular drawn on lead I axis through +10.

Step IV

Now calculate the net deflection in lead aVF in the same manner. In the given ECG, the net deflection is –12 [–13+ (+1) = –12]. Now plot –12 in the lead axis of lead aVF as shown in Fig. 3.19.

Step V

Draw a perpendicular through the plotted point on lead aVF axis and prolong it to meet the perpendicular drawn on lead I axis as shown in Fig. 3.20.

Step VI

Draw a line joining the point of the intersection of axis of lead I and aVF and the point of intersection of the two perpendicular lines. The QRS axis is –55° as shown in Fig. 3.21.

The various causes of right and left axis deviation are summarized in Box 3.1.

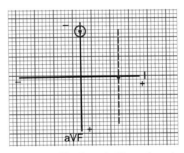

Fig. 3.19 Plotting of –12 on the axis of lead aVF.

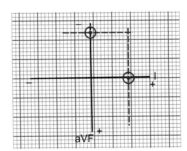

Fig. 3.20 Perpendicular drawn on axis of lead aVF through –12.

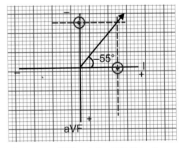

Fig. 3.21 QRS axis is –55°. This shows that the exact calculated axis is –55° (left axis deviation).

Box 3.1   Causes of Right and Left Axis Deviation

Right Axis Deviation
- Right ventricular hypertrophy
- Chronic obstructive pulmonary disease
- Right bundle branch block
- Left posterior hemiblock
- Pulmonary embolism
- Dextrocardia
- Anterolateral myocardial infarction
- Wolff–Parkinson–White (WPW) syndrome
- Normal variant
- Left pneumothorax

Left Axis Deviation
- Left ventricular hypertrophy
- Left anterior hemiblock
- Inferior wall myocardial infarction
- Emphysema
- WPW syndrome
- Normal variant

BIBLIOGRAPHY

1. Burger HC and van Millan JB. Heart-vector and leads. Part II. *Br Heart J* 1947; 9(3), 154–160.
2. Dougherty JD. The relation of the frontal plane QRS axis to the anatomic position of the heart. *J Electrocardiol* 1970; 3(3–4), 267–284.
3. Durakovic Z and Mimica M. Left axis deviation and tall R waves in the electrocardiogram. *J Electrocardiol* 1981; 14(1), 31–37.
4. Grant RP. The relationship between the anatomic position of the heart and the electrocardiogram; a criticism of unipolar electrocardiography. *Circulation* 1953; 7(6), 890–902.
5. Hakki AH, Anderson GJ, Iskandrian AS, et al. A simple method to determine the electrocardiographic frontal plane axis. *J Electrocardiol* 1982; 15(3), 285–288.

6. Schamroth L. *An Introduction to Electrocardiography*, Seventh edition, Blackwell Science (Indian Reprint), 2002; pp. 34–48.
7. Dubin S and Staib J. Annotation: numerical calculation of the mean electrical axis of electrocardiographic deflections. *J Electrocardiol* 1977; 10(1), 77–78.
8. Meek S and Morris F. ABC of clinical electrocardiography. Introduction. I-leads, rate, rhythm, and cardiac axis. *BMJ* 2002; 324(7334), 415–418.

CHAPTER 4

Normal ECG Variants

Chapter Outline

INTRODUCTION

The electrocardiogram (ECG) tracings that appear to be abnormal yet occur in normal healthy persons are called variants of normal ECG. These tracings depend on age, sex, body mass index, position of heart, race, heavy meal, exercise, etc. Some of the normal variants can be recognized easily and are given certain names such as persistent juvenile pattern, early repolarization syndrome.

WELL-RECOGNIZED VARIANTS OF A NORMAL ECG

Early Repolarization Syndrome

Early repolarization syndrome is characterized by S–T segment elevation. It is a common variant and is often confused with myocardial infarction and pericarditis. The S–T segment elevation may be up to 5 mm but it is usually about 2–3 mm. The S–T segment is concave upwards (in contrast to myocardial infarction) and is more prominent in leads V4–V6. Serial ECG recordings do not show any evolutionary changes as observed in myocardial infarction (Fig. 4.1). The ECG manifestations are the following:

1. Concave upwards S–T segment elevation
2. Prominent J waves (J waves are junctional waves, i.e., at the junction of QRS complex and S–T segment)

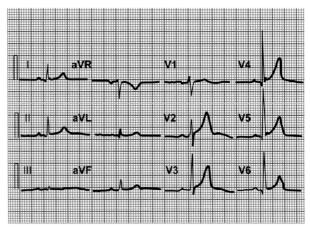

Fig. 4.1 Early repolarization syndrome. This electrocardiogram is taken from a 40-year-old man who presented with chest pain. Note the concave upwards S–T segment elevation in leads V4–V6. Also note the prominent J waves in leads V4 and V5. This type of ECG is often confused with S–T segment elevation of myocardial infarction.

3. Tall R waves in leads V4–V6
4. Tall and symmetrical T waves
5. Narrow q waves in leads V4–V6

Persistent Juvenile Pattern
In infancy and childhood, the T wave is normally inverted in leads V1–V4 and if these changes persist in adulthood, then it is known as persistent juvenile pattern (Fig. 4.2).

Non-Specific T Wave Changes
Often we come across persons in whom the T waves are inverted and detailed examination and investigation do not reveal any anatomical or pathological changes in the heart. They are normal persons in whom the T waves are normally inverted. The T waves may also be inverted in the following conditions:

1. After heavy meal
2. After hyperventilation
3. As a response to anxiety and fear

Anxiety and Hyperventilation States
Anxiety and hyperventilation often cause changes in ECG in normal persons who do not suffer from any cardiac disease. These changes

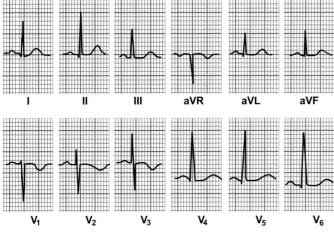

Fig. 4.2   Persistent juvenile pattern.

are thought to be due to autonomic imbalance. The various abnormalities detected are:

1. Sinus tachycardia
2. Prolongation of P–R interval
3. S–T segment depression with or without T wave inversion especially in inferior leads

Heavy Carbohydrate Meal

ECG changes are known to occur in healthy individuals after a meal rich in carbohydrates. The changes are thought to occur due to carbohydrate-mediated changes in potassium level, and it is considered to be a physiological condition. The main changes in ECG are S–T segment depression and T wave inversion.

BIBLIOGRAPHY

1. Assali AR, Khamaysi N and Birnbaum Y. Juvenile ECG pattern in adult black Arabs. *J Electrocardiol* 1997; 30(2), 87–90.
2. Bachman S, Sparrow D and Smith LK. Effect of aging on the electrocardiogram. *Am J Cardiol* 1981; 48, 513–516.
3. Fenichel NN. A long term study of concave RS-T elevation—a normal variant of the electrocardiogram. *Angiology* 1962; 13, 360–366.
4. Schamroth L. *An Introduction to Electrocardiography*, Seventh edition, Blackwell Science (Indian Reprint), UK, 2002; pp. 125–128.
5. Liebman J. The early repolarization syndrome is a variation of normal. *J Electrocardiol* 2007; 40(5), 391.
6. Littmann D. Persistence of the juvenile pattern in the precordial leads of healthy adult Negroes, with report of electrocardiographic survey on 300 Negroes and 200 white subjects. *Am Heart J* 1946; 32, 370.

CHAPTER 5

Atrial and Ventricular Hypertrophy

There may be hypertrophy or enlargement of atria, ventricles or both. *Dilatation* usually means an increase in the internal diameter and *hypertrophy* usually means thickening of the muscular wall. The term *enlargement* is usually used for atria and hypertrophy is used for ventricles.

In atrial enlargement the changes are mainly seen in P waves whereas in ventricular hypertrophy the changes are mainly seen in QRS complexes.

ATRIAL ENLARGEMENT

Atrial enlargement/hypertrophy occurs in conditions like chronic obstructive pulmonary disease, rheumatic heart disease or congenital heart disease with pulmonary hypertension etc. In a child, the most probable cause of atrial enlargement is a congenital heart disease. Atrial enlargement is mainly manifested by changes in P waves.

Right Atrial Enlargement

Right atrial enlargement/hypertrophy is commonly seen in mitral stenosis, cor pulmonale, atrial septal defect (ASD), tricuspid stenosis, pulmonary stenosis, tricuspid regurgitation etc. The right atrial enlargement has the following electrocardiogram (ECG) changes:

1. *P pulmonale*: It is reflected by the presence of tall- and peaked P waves in leads II, III and aVF. The amplitude is more than 2.5 mm. It is called *P pulmonale* because it occurs frequently due to pulmonary hypertension (Fig. 5.1a, b).

2. P wave in lead V1 may be normal or biphasic with a slight increase in amplitude (>1.5 mm) of the initial component.

3. P wave axis is deviated to right (between +80° and +90°). The normal P wave axis is around +60°.

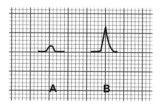

Left Atrial Enlargement

Left atrial enlargement/hypertrophy is often seen as secondary to left ventricular hypertrophy (LVH) in hypertensive heart disease, cardiomyopathy, aortic stenosis, mitral

Fig. 5.1a Diagram of normal- and tall P waves of right atrial enlargement. Note the round contour of normal P wave (A) and the tall- and peaked contour of P wave of right atrial enlargement (B). The height of P wave of right atrial enlargement is more than 2.5 mm.

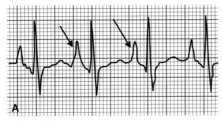

Lead II

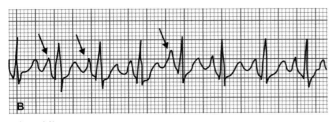

Lead II

Fig. 5.1b P pulmonale. (A) This ECG is recorded from a 54-year-old man suffering from cor pulmonale due to COPD. Note the tall- and peaked P waves (arrow). (B) This ECG is recorded from a 46-year-old woman suffering from pulmonary hypertension due to idiopathic pulmonary fibrosis. Note the tall- and peaked P waves (arrow).

regurgitation, ventricular septal defect (VSD) etc. Left atrial enlargement is characterized by:

1. *P mitrale*: This is a wide, double-peaked, prolonged P wave. This is best seen in lead II. The P wave duration is prolonged to greater than 0.11 s. This is due to the delay of the left atrial component of the P wave. The duration between the two peaks of P wave is greater than 0.04 s (Figs. 5.2 and 5.3). It is commonly seen in mitral stenosis.

2. The P wave in lead V1 is biphasic with a deep, wide, terminal negative component. P terminal force (Morris Index, for evaluation of terminal negative component) is calculated by multiplying the depth of the negative component (in mm) by the duration of the negative component (in second). It is expressed in mms. Normally it is less than 0.03 mms. P terminal force is greater than 0.03 mms represents left atrial enlargement (Fig. 5.4).

3. Left axis deviation of P wave. The P wave axis is directed between +45° and –30°.

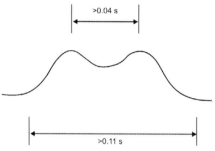

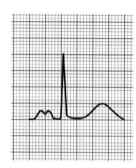

Fig. 5.2   Diagram of P mitrale. The total duration of a P wave is more than 0.11 s and the interval between the two peaks of P wave is more than 0.04 s.

Fig. 5.3   P mitrale. Note the bifid P wave.

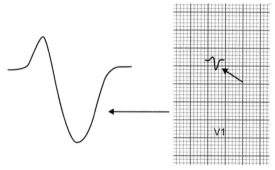

Fig. 5.4   Diagram of P wave of left atrial enlargement in lead V1. Note the deep, wide negative component of the biphasic P wave (arrow).

Combined Left and Right Atrial Enlargement

There are certain conditions in which both the atria are enlarged together. The conditions are mentioned in Box 5.1.

Box 5.1   Conditions Associated with Biatrial Enlargement

- Mitral stenosis with severe pulmonary hypertension
- Mitral stenosis with tricuspid stenosis
- Mitral stenosis with tricuspid regurgitation
- Lutembacher's syndrome i.e., ASD with acquired rheumatic mitral stenosis
- ASD

The ECG features of combined left and right atrial enlargement/ hypertrophy are the following:

1. The P wave will be wide and notched with an increased amplitude. When such type of P wave is associated with an initial component that is taller than the terminal component then it is known as *P tricuspidale*. It is commonly seen in tricuspid valve diseases and may be seen in frontal plane leads.
2. In lead V1 there will be a biphasic P wave in which the initial component is tall and peaked and the terminal component is wide, deep and delayed. The initial component represents right atrial enlargement and the terminal component represents the left atrial enlargement.

VENTRICULAR HYPERTROPHY

Ventricular hypertrophy occurs due to systolic or volume overload of ventricles. Systolic overload leads to concentric hypertrophy in which there is an increase in thickness of wall but the diameter of the chamber of ventricle does not increase significantly. In volume overload there is an increase in wall thickness but there is a significant increase in the diameter of the ventricular chamber too.

Left Ventricular Hypertrophy

The various causes of LVH are mentioned in Box 5.2.

The following are the ECG changes of LVH due to systolic overload (excess resistance to outflow of blood from left ventricle), for example, in aortic stenosis or hypertension:

1. Abnormalities of QRS complex
2. Abnormalities of S–T segment and T wave

Box 5.2   Some Important Causes of LVH

- Aortic stenosis or aortic regurgitation
- Hypertensive heart disease
- Mitral regurgitation
- Congenital heart disease like patent ductus arteriosus (PDA), coarctation of aorta, tricuspid atresia, etc
- Hypertrophic cardiomyopathy

3. Abnormalities of QRS axis
4. Inversion of U wave
5. Left atrial enlargement

Abnormalities of QRS Complex
Increased amplitude of QRS complex

Hypertrophy means an increase in the thickness of the wall of a ventricle (Fig. 5.5a). As ventricular activation occurs from endocardium to epicardium, the amplitude of the R and S waves indicates the thickness of the ventricular wall. The amplitude of the QRS complex is increased in LVH. There is a deep S wave in lead V1 and a tall R wave in leads V5 and V6. In an adult above 35 years of age, if the sum of R wave in lead V5 and the depth of S wave in lead V1 exceeds 35 mm, it indicates LVH (Fig. 5.5b). Whenever one suspects LVH, then he/she must look for this criterion in the very beginning itself. Sokolow–Lyon voltage criteria used for the diagnosis of LVH are given in Box 5.3.

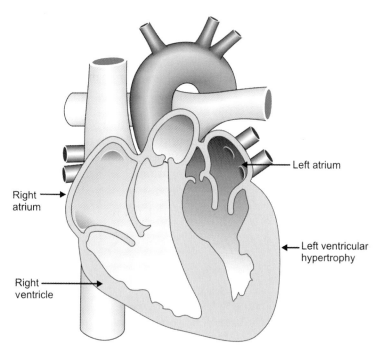

Right
atrium

Right
ventricle

Left atrium

Left ventricular
hypertrophy

Fig. 5.5a   Left ventricular hypertrophy. Note the wall thickness of left ventricle and the small left ventricular cavity.

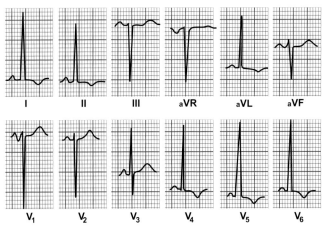

Fig. 5.5b   Left ventricular hypertrophy. This ECG is recorded from a 60-year-old patient suffering from hypertension for 17 years. SV1 + RV5 is 37 mm. There are tall R waves in leads I and aVL. Note the S–T segment and T wave change in leads V4, V5 and V6.

Box 5.3   Sokolow–Lyon Voltage Criteria for LVH Diagnosis

- RI + SIII ≥ 2.5 mV (25 mm)
- R in aVL >1.2 mV (12 mm)
- R in aVF >2.0 mV (20 mm)
- S in V1 >2.4 mV (24 mm)
- R in V5 and V6 >2.6 mV (26 mm)
- R in V5 or V6 + S in V1 >3.5 mV (35 mm)

Increase in ventricular activation time (VAT)

VAT is very prominently increased in LVH due to systolic overload. It is an indirect measurement of the time taken by an impulse to travel from endo- to epicardium and hence it is often increased in LVH to more than 0.05 s in lead V5 or V6.

Counterclockwise electric rotation

The counterclockwise electric rotation of heart is reflected by shifting of transition zone to lead V3 or even lead V2.

Abnormalities of S–T Segment and T Wave

In LVH the LV is under strain due to ischaemia and is manifested by S–T segment depression and T wave inversion in leads V5, V6, aVL and lead I. The S–T segment depression is usually mild with a slight upward convexity.

Abnormalities of QRS Axis

Early- and uncomplicated LVH is associated with normal QRS axis; but the long-standing LVH, especially that associated with hypertension, may lead to fibrosis, which may, in turn, affect the left-anterior fascicle resulting in left-anterior hemiblock and thus results in left axis deviation.

Inversion of U Wave

There may be an inversion of U wave in the left-sided chest leads. It is more commonly seen in diastolic overload like aortic incompetence.

Left Atrial Enlargement

Left atrial enlargement provides a contributory evidence of LVH. It helps in the diagnosis of LVH in the presence of left bundle branch block. There may be a wide, notched P wave in lead II and a biphasic P wave in lead V1, with a deep negative component.

Combining all the above-mentioned criteria, there is a scoring system called Romhilt–Estes point score (Box 5.4). LVH is indicated if this score is 5 or more. These criteria are applicable mainly for LVH due to systolic overload. All the diagnostic criteria of LVH are summarized in Box 5.5.

Box 5.4   Romhilt–Estes Point Score

- Increased QRS voltage: 3 points
- S–T and T changes: 3 points
- P wave of LAE: 3 points
- LAD: 2 points
- Increased VAT: 1 point

Box 5.5   Diagnostic Criteria for LVH

- Increased amplitude of QRS complex
- Increase in VAT in lead V5 or V6
- Counterclockwise rotation of heart
- S–T and T-strain pattern in lead V5 or V6
- LAD
- Inversion of U wave
- LAE
- Romhilt–Estes point of 5 or more

LVH due to diastolic overload (excess blood flow in left ventricle) as happens in aortic incompetence or mitral incompetence has the following features:

1. Like in the systolic overload there are tall R waves in leads V5 and V6 also. They may be even more tall in the diastolic overload than the way they are seen in the systolic overload.
2. There are narrow, deep Q waves in leads V5 and V6. They do not indicate any old myocardial infarction.
3. The T waves in leads V5 and V6 are taller than the normal T waves seen in those leads. Often they are pointed with an arrowhead appearance.
4. The S–T segment in leads V5 and V6 are slightly elevated with concavity upwards (Fig. 5.6).

Right Ventricular Hypertrophy

Right ventricular hypertrophy (RVH) is seen in various conditions like cor pulmonale, mitral stenosis, tricuspid incompetence, tetralogy of fallot, pulmonary stenosis, idiopathic pulmonary hypertension etc. (Fig. 5.7). ECG changes of RVH are much less common when compared with LVH.

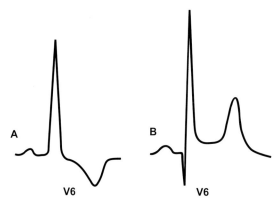

Fig. 5.6 Diagram showing LVH in a systolic (A) and a diastolic (B) overload. In a systolic overload, the initial q wave often disappears whereas in a diastolic overload, the initial q wave becomes prominent. The amplitude of R wave is increased in both. The T wave is inverted with S–T segment depression in systolic overload, but in diastolic overload the S–T segment may be minimally elevated with upward concavity.

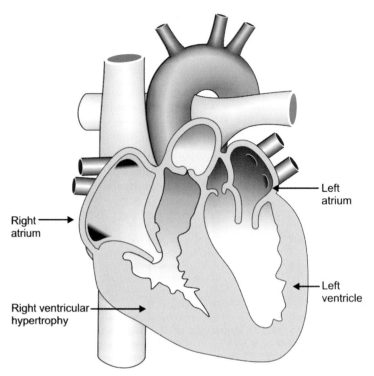

Right
atrium

Left
atrium

Left
ventricle

Right ventricular
hypertrophy

Fig. 5.7   Right ventricular hypertrophy (RVH). Note the thickness of right ventricular wall and the decrease in cavity size. This is concentric hypertrophy.

RVH is characterized by the following abnormalities:

1. Abnormality of QRS complex
2. Abnormality of S–T segment and T wave
3. Abnormality of QRS axis
4. Right atrial enlargement

Abnormality of QRS Complex
Dominance of R wave in the right-sided chest leads

In RVH the R wave in V1 becomes prominent when compared with S wave. The rS complex gradually changes to RS, Rs, R and then qR complexes. There is a gradual increase in the height of R wave and diminution of S wave. This is expressed as R:S ratio. If the ratio exceeds 1 then RVH is diagnosed (Fig. 5.8). One must look for this feature in the beginning if there is suspicion of RVH. The S waves

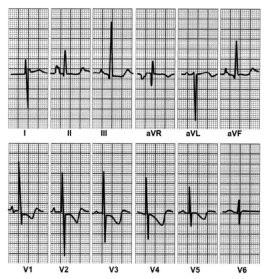

Fig. 5.8 Right ventricular hypertrophy (RVH). This ECG is recorded from a 25-year-old female suffering from mitral stenosis with pulmonary hypertension. The features of RVH are tall R wave in lead V1 with S–T segment and T wave changes. S–T segment and T wave changes are present in the right-sided chest leads. Clockwise rotation of heart is observed with the transition zone shifted in lead V6. There are features of biatrial enlargement with right axis deviation of QRS axis.

are prominent in leads V5 and V6. The amplitude of R wave is more than 5 mm in lead V1. Always remember that there are several other causes too for the tall R wave seen in lead V1; that is, posterior wall myocardial infarction, persistent juvenile pattern, RBBB, dextrocardia, WPW (Wolff–Parkinson–White) syndrome, etc.

Increase in VAT in lead V1

There is an increase in VAT (>0.02 s) in lead V1. This is because more time is taken by the impulse to travel through the hypertrophied right ventricular free wall.

Clockwise electric rotation

The transition zone may be shifted to lead V5 or V6. All the chest leads may show prominent R waves only.

Right bundle branch block

RBBB is often associated with RVH. It may be complete or incomplete (Fig. 5.9).

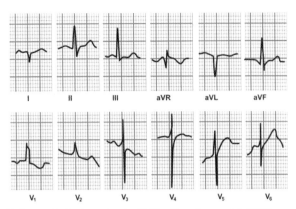

Fig. 5.9   Right ventricular hypertrophy (RVH) with an incomplete RBBB.

Abnormalities of S–T Segment and T Wave

A strain pattern is seen in the right-sided chest leads. The S–T segment is slightly depressed with a slight convexity upwards. Inversion of T waves is seen in leads V1–V4. Sometimes, they may appear deep and pointed too. The U wave may sometimes appear inverted in leads V1 and V2.

Abnormalities of QRS Axis

There is right axis deviation of QRS axis. The QRS axis lies between +110° and +180°. Sometimes it is the only feature of RVH. The axis may rarely be deviated to the right superior quadrant that is, northwest axis.

Right Atrial Enlargement

ECG evidence of right atrial enlargement is often associated with RVH. The T waves become tall and pointed in lead II. The diagnostic criteria of RVH are summarized in Box 5.6.

Box 5.6   Diagnostic Criteria for RVH

- R:S ratio greater than 1 in lead V1
- Increase in VAT in lead V1 or V2
- Clockwise rotation of heart
- Right axis deviation
- S–T and T-strain pattern in leads V1–V4
- Right atrial enlargement

Box. 5.7   Causes of Biventricular Hypertrophy

- Dilated cardiomyopathy
- Congenital heart disease: Eisenmenger's syndrome
- Multiple valvular lesions

Biventricular Hypertrophy

There are certain conditions in which both the ventricles are hypertrophied. The various conditions are mentioned in Box 5.7.

The combined right and left ventricular hypertrophy is manifested with the following features:

1. ECG features of LVH are associated with right axis deviation.
2. ECG features of LVH are associated with clockwise rotation, that is, transition zone in lead V5 or V6.
3. ECG features of LVH are associated with tall R wave in lead V1 especially if R:S ratio is greater than 1.
4. Katz–Wachtel phenomenon: large biphasic complexes in lead V2 or V3.
5. P mitrale with R:S ratio greater than 1 in lead V1 or right QRS axis deviation.

BIBLIOGRAPHY

1. Benchimol A, Reich F and Desser KB. Comparison of the electrocardiogram and vectorcardiogram for the diagnosis of left atrial enlargement. *J Electrocardiol* 1976; 9(3), 215–218.
2. Pewsner D, Jüni P, Egger M, Battaglia M, Sundström J, Bachmann LM. Accuracy of electrocardiography in diagnosis of left ventricular hypertrophy in arterial hypertension: systematic review. *BMJ*; 2007;335(7622), 711.
3. Eren N and Ilerigelen B. Diagnostic value of electrocardiogram for left ventricular hypertrophy in elderly patients with hypertension. *J Electrocardiol* 2007; 40(4), S57.
4. Leo S. An Introduction to Electrocardiography, Seventh edition, Blackwell Science Indian Reprint, 2002; pp. 67–85.

5. Marriott HJL and Wagner GS. Marriott's Practical Electrocardiography. Hagerstwon, MD: Lippincott Williams & Wilkins, 2001.

6. Martynova E, Kuznetsov V, Solovyev V, et al. Automated computer analysis in diagnostics of left ventricular hypertrophy by electrocardiography. *J Electrocardiol* 2007; 40(4), S41–S42.

7. Ristow B and Schiller NB. Detecting left atrial enlargement by ECG—a comparison of 4 methods. *J Electrocardiol* 2006; 39(2), 230–231.

CHAPTER 6

Conduction Disturbances

SINOATRIAL BLOCK

In sinoatrial block (SA block) the impulse is blocked at the junction of SA node and atrial myocardium. Therefore, the atrial and ventricular activation does not occur and as a result a complete PQRST complex is not recorded (Fig. 6.1).

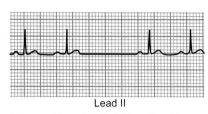

Lead II

Fig. 6.1 Sinoatrial block. Note that after two normal complexes there is a drop of entire PQRS complex followed by normal rhythm.

SA block is commonly a manifestation of increased vagal tone. It may be seen in normal persons also. Other important causes are carotid sinus pressure, drug toxicity (quinidine, digitalis) or in diseases involving the SA nodal area. It can be a feature of sick sinus syndrome. The various causes of SA block are summarized in Box 6.1.

ATRIOVENTRICULAR BLOCK

Atrioventricular (AV) block is the disturbance in conduction of atrial impulse through the AV conducting system, i.e., the AV node, the bundle of His or His-Purkinje system. It can result from either a functional or pathological defect in the atria, AV node, bundle of His, or bundle branches. The functional block may be due to increased vagal tone. There are three degrees of block.

Box 6.1   Causes of Sinoatrial Block
• Digitalis toxicity
• Young athletes
• Uraemia
• Hypokalaemia
• Rheumatic fever
• Sick sinus syndrome
• Acute myocardial infarction
• Myocarditis
• Carotid sinus sensitivity

1. First degree of AV block: Delay in conduction.
2. Second degree of AV block: Intermittent interruption in conduction.
3. Third degree or complete AV block: Complete interruption in conduction.

First-degree AV Block

First-degree AV block may occur in the absence of any cardiac disease. There is a delay in conduction of every impulse through the AV conducting system (Fig. 6.2a). As a result, there is a prolongation of P–R interval above 0.20 s in every PQRS complex (Fig. 6.2b, c).

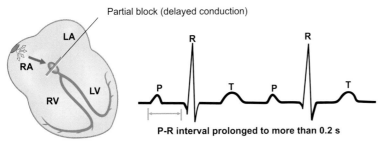

Fig. 6.2a   First-degree atrioventricular (AV) block.

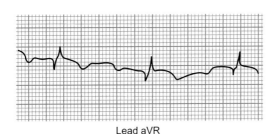

Lead aVR

Fig. 6.2b   First-degree AV block. In this electrocardiogram, the P–R interval is 0.32 s. This patient was taking atenolol (beta-blocker) for hypertension. In this case, the P–R interval becomes normal after stopping atenolol.

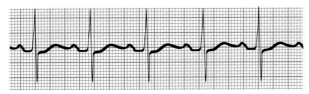

Fig. 6.2c   First-degree AV block. The P–R interval is 0.24 s.

The rhythm is regular without any dropped beat. All the beats are conducted to the ventricles, i.e., every P wave is followed by a QRS complex. The various causes of first-degree AV block are summarized in Box 6.2.

Second-degree AV Block

Second-degree AV block is usually due to organic heart disease. Second-degree AV block is characterized by intermittent interruption of AV conduction. In this condition, some of the impulses are conducted while the others are not conducted to the ventricles. The P wave is not followed by the QRS complex, as the ventricles are not depolarized. The second-degree AV block may be constant or variable.

The various causes of second-degree AV block are summarized in Box 6.3.

There are two types of second-degree AV block: Mobitz type I and Mobitz type II.

Box 6.2   Causes of First-degree Atrioventricular Block

- Coronary artery disease
- Rheumatic fever
- Digitalis toxicity
- Drugs—beta-blocker, quinidine
- Atrial septal defect
- Ebstein's anomaly
- Increased vagal tone
- Hyperkalaemia
- Idiopathic

Box 6.3   Causes of Second-degree Atrioventricular Block

- Digitalis toxicity
- Rheumatic carditis
- Coronary heart disease
- Diphtheria myocarditis
- In the presence of atrial fibrillation and flutter (physiological)
- Beta-blocker and verapamil toxicity
- Increased vagal tone
- Hyperkalaemia

Mobitz Type I (Wenckebach) AV Block

The conduction of impulse through the AV conducting system becomes increasingly difficult and ultimately an impulse fails to conduct to the ventricles. The first atrial impulse produces a complex with a normal P–R interval. This is followed by gradual prolongation of P–R interval in successive beats followed by dropping of a QRS complex. This means one has to look for gradual prolongation of P–R interval followed by a P wave and absence of QRS complex (replaced by a pause). After this, the AV conduction system recovers and the sequence is repeated in a cyclic manner (Fig. 6.3). The number of beats in each cycle may not be constant. Usual site of block is at the AV node.

Mobitz Type II AV Block

In Mobitz type II AV block, there is no gradual prolongation of P–R interval. There is regular or irregular interruption of conduction through AV conducting system (Fig. 6.4a). For a specified number of P waves, the number of QRS complexes is less, e.g., if the number of P waves is 2 and the number of QRS complexes is 1 then the block will be 2:1 AV block (Fig. 6.4b). If every second P wave is not followed by the QRS complex (2:1 AV block) or if after every third P wave there is one QRS complex (3:1 AV block), then the heart rate will be regular but in irregular or variable AV block the heart rhythm will be irregular.

Usual site of block is in the His-Purkinje system. Atrial rhythm is regular. Ventricular rhythm is irregular (regular in 2:1 AV block).

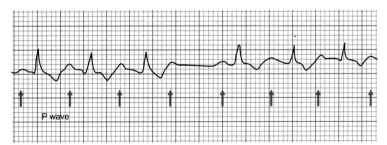

Fig. 6.3 Wenckebach phenomenon. This electrocardiogram was recorded from a 14-year-old patient suffering from acute rheumatic carditis. This conduction disturbance became normal with the treatment of rheumatic fever. Note the gradual prolongation of P–R interval in the first three QRS complexes, which are followed by a P wave with the loss of QRS complex. After this, there is a recovery of conduction and there is a normal P–R interval followed by gradual prolongation of the P–R interval.

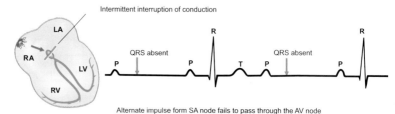

Fig. 6.4a   Mobitz type II atrioventricular (AV) block.

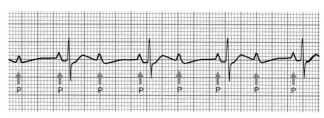

Fig. 6.4b   2:1 AV block. Note that after every normal complex there is a P wave, which is not followed by a QRS complex. So, there are two P waves and one QRS complex and thus the block is 2:1 AV block.

P waves are normal in shape and size. P–R interval is within normal limits. QRS complex duration is usually ≥ 0.10 s but they are periodically absent after the P waves.

Third-Degree AV Block (Complete AV Block)

Third-degree AV block is also called complete heart block. It is characterized by complete and permanent failure of conduction through AV conducting system (Fig. 6.5a). The block may occur at the AV node, bundle of His or bundle branches. The ventricles are activated by an ectopic pacemaker situated either in AV node junction below the block or in the ventricles. Thus, two different pacemakers activate the atria and the ventricles and the two rhythms are asynchronous. Therefore, there is atrioventricular dissociation (Fig. 6.5b, c).

The EGG manifestations are the following:

1. AV dissociation: P wave and QRS complex bears no relationship with each other.
2. Slow ventricular rate: The ventricular rate is slow and usually in the range of 30–35 beats/min. The atrial rate is greater than the ventricular rate and the atrial and ventricular rhythms are regular.

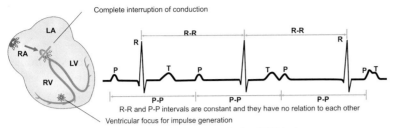

Fig. 6.5a   Complete atrioventricular (AV) block.

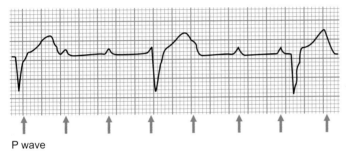

P wave

Fig. 6.5b   Complete AV block. This electrocardiogram was recorded from a 67-year-old man suffering from acute myocardial infarction. Note that there is no correlation between the P waves and the QRS complexes. This means that the atria and the ventricles are activated by two different pacemakers (atrioventricular dissociation). The wide and bizarre QRS complex with slow ventricular rate suggests that the ventricular pacemaker is situated in the ventricular myocardium. If it was situated in the bundle of His or in the bundle branches, then the QRS complexes would have been narrow with higher ventricular rate.

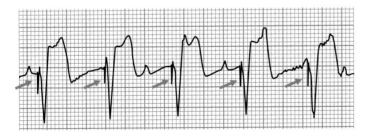

Fig. 6.5c   The same patient of Fig. 6.5b was treated with temporary pacemaker. Note the increase in the ventricular rate and the pacemaker spikes (arrow) that precede each QRS complex. The QRS complexes have widened because the pacemaker activates the ventricular myocardium and the impulse does not travel through the normal conducting system.

3. QRS configuration: If the ectopic pacemaker is situated in the AV junction or in the bundle of His proximal to the bundle branches, then the QRS configuration is normal or near normal but if the pacemaker is situated in the Purkinje fibres or in the myocardium then the QRS complexes become broad, slanted and bizarre in shape. The various causes of complete AV block are summarized in Box 6.4.

How to Interpret the Three Degrees of AV Block?

To identify the three degrees of block, the most important thing is P–R interval. By measuring the P–R interval and following the steps mentioned below, the three different degrees of block can be identified.

Step I

First, see whether the P–R interval is fixed or varying from one complex to other in the rhythm strip.

Step II

If the P–R interval is fixed in all the complexes in the rhythm strip then it is either first-degree AV block or Mobitz type II second-degree AV block.

Step III

To differentiate between them calculate the P–R interval correctly. If it is prolonged (more than 0.2 s) in all the leads then it is first-degree AV block.

Box 6.4   Causes of Complete Atrioventricular Block

- Congenital complete atrioventricular block
- Coronary artery disease
- Intracardiac surgery
- Congenital heart disease: Corrected transposition of the great vessels, ventricular septal defect, ostium primum type of atrial septal defect.
- Lenegre's disease, Lev's disease
- Drugs—digitalis, quinidine
- Amyloid heart disease
- Myocarditis and endocarditis
- Acute rheumatic carditis
- Miscellaneous—Chagas disease, intracardiac tubercle, gumma, granuloma, tumour

Step IV

If the P–R interval is normal but there are certain complexes in which the P wave is present but the QRS complex is absent and it is not possible to calculate P–R interval in them, then it is Mobitz type II second-degree AV block.

Step V

If P–R interval is varying then think about Mobitz type I second-degree AV block and third-degree AV block.

Step VI

To differentiate between the two see whether all the P–R intervals are different or there is progressive increase in the P–R interval.

Step VII

If there is progressive increase in the P–R interval, then it is Mobitz type I second-degree AV block.

Step VIII

If all the P–R intervals are varying, then it is third-degree AV block (this is, however, not the true P–R interval, as there is no conduction of impulse from the atria to the ventricle).

Step IX

After following these primary steps look for all the other features of AV block as already mentioned and come to a definite diagnosis.

Algorithm for Interpretation of Various Types of AV Block

Rhythm strip electrocardiogram (ECG) (Lead II)

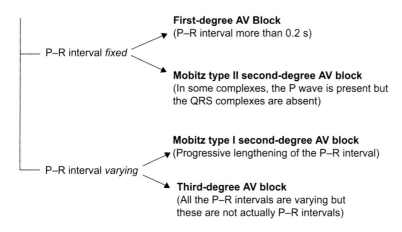

INTRAVENTRICULAR CONDUCTION DEFECT

Intraventricular conduction defect means abnormality of conduction through the intraventricular conduction system distal to bundle of His. The block may be at the level of right bundle branch, left bundle branch, left anterior fascicle, left posterior fascicle, or at the level of peripheral Purkinje fibres.

BUNDLE BRANCH BLOCK

Bundle branch block means partial or complete failure of the impulse to travel through either the left or the right or both the bundle branches. Mainly there are two types of bundle branch blocks, i.e., right and left bundle branch blocks, which will be discussed here (Fig. 6.6).

Right Bundle Branch Block

Right bundle branch block (RBBB) is characterized by delay or interruption in conduction of impulse through the right bundle branch (Fig. 6.7a). RBBB is a common ECG finding and alone it is not suggestive of any disease, because it is frequently present in normal persons also. Acute exacerbation of chronic obstructive pulmonary disease or acute pulmonary embolism can lead to a transient RBBB. It may be a rate-related phenomenon also. The various causes of RBBB are

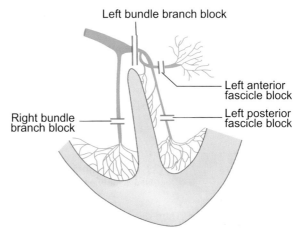

Fig. 6.6   Diagram of bundle branch blocks.

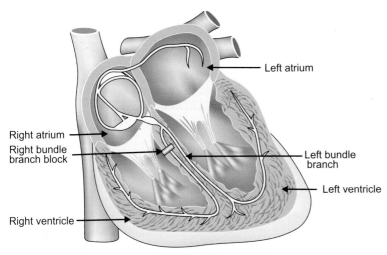

Fig. 6.7a   Right bundle branch block.

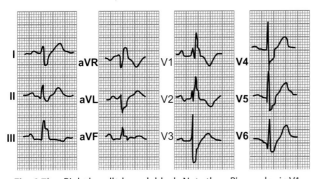

Fig. 6.7b   Right bundle branch block. Note the rsR' complex in V1.

summarized in Box 6.5. The ECG manifestations of complete RBBB are the following:

1. Wide, slurred QRS complex in lead V1 or V2 with rsR' or rSR' pattern (Figs. 6.7b and 6.8).
2. The duration of QRS complex is ≥ 0.12 s. According to some authorities, the duration should be ≥ 0.14 s.
3. S–T segment depression and T wave inversion in lead V1 or V2.

Box 6.5   Causes of Right Bundle Branch Block

- Normally present without heart disease
- Coronary artery disease
- Cardiomyopathies
- Atrial septal defect (ostium primum type)
- Acute massive pulmonary embolism
- Associated with right ventricular hypertrophy
- Ebstein's anomaly
- Congenital
- Cardiac contusion
- Idiopathic

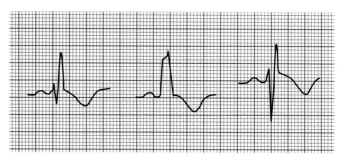

Fig. 6.8   Types of rsR' complexes in lead V1.

4. Ventricular activation time (VAT) is more than 0.06 s in lead V1 or V2.
5. Wide-slurred S wave in leads I, aVL, V5 and V6.
6. There is a small r wave in lead V1 and a small q wave in lead V6.

Incomplete RBBB

In incomplete RBBB, the QRS duration is not prolonged beyond 0.11 s and the VAT in lead V1 is less than 0.06 s. There is diminution of S wave in lead V2 with slurring in the upstroke of S wave and it is the earliest feature of incomplete RBBB. Diminution of S wave may be the only feature of incomplete RBBB sometimes.

Left Bundle Branch Block

Left bundle branch block (LBBB) is characterized by delay or complete block of transmission of impulse through the left bundle

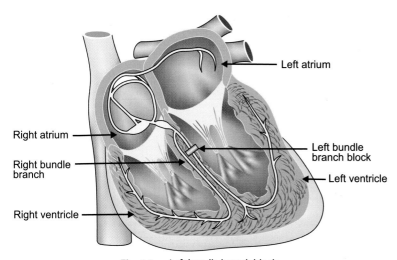

Fig. 6.9a   Left bundle branch block.

branch (Fig. 6.9a). The delay produces incomplete LBBB and the complete block produces complete LBBB.

LBBB may be found in almost any type of cardiac disease and it always indicates some organic heart disease unlike RBBB. It may be commonly observed in conditions that cause left ventricular hypertrophy such as hypertension or aortic stenosis. It is uncommon in congenital heart disease. LBBB may be transient or permanent in the same tracing or in serial tracings. Transient LBBB occurs after myocardial infarction or after consumption of drugs such as digitalis, acute myocarditis, heart failure. Permanent LBBB indicates organic heart disease. LBBB may be related to heart rate. The various causes of LBBB are summarized in Box 6.6. The ECG manifestations of complete LBBB are the following:

1. There is wide, slurred, bizarre QRS complex in lead V5 or V6 with rsR' pattern (M pattern) (Fig. 6.9b; also see Fig. 6.10).
2. VAT is prolonged to more than 0.09 s in lead V5 or V6.
3. Q or q wave is absent in lead V5 or V6. Presence of q wave signifies myocardial infarction.
4. QRS duration is more than 0.12 s.
5. The S–T segment and T wave are directed opposite to the QRS deflection. Therefore, in lead V5 or lead V6, S–T segment is depressed and the T wave is inverted. Complete LBBB often mimics anterior wall myocardial infarction.

Box 6.6   Causes of Left Bundle Branch Block

- Coronary artery disease
- Cardiomyopathies
- Myocarditis
- Hypertensive heart disease
- Aortic valve disease

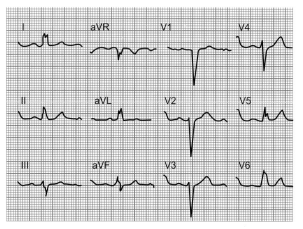

Fig. 6.9b   Left bundle branch block. This electrocardiogram is taken from a 62-year-old man suffering from long-standing hypertension with coronary artery disease. Note the widening of QRS complex and the notching of the R wave in leads I, aVL, V5, and V6. The classical 'M' pattern is seen in lead V5.

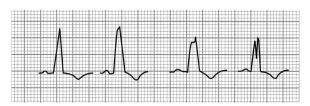

Fig. 6.10   Types of rsR' complexes in lead V6.

Incomplete LBBB

In incomplete LBBB, there is delayed conduction through the left bundle. The features of incomplete LBBB are the following:

1. Small q wave in lead V5 or V6 disappears and there is a tall R wave.
2. Small r wave in lead V1 disappears and there is a big QS complex.

3. Gradually the other features of complete LBBB appear, but the width of QRS complex is less than 0.12 s and VAT is less than 0.09 s.

DIVISIONAL (FASCICULAR) BLOCKS

The left bundle divides into two fascicles: anterior and posterior fascicles. The anterior fascicle spreads over the anterosuperior endocardial surface of the left ventricle. The posterior fascicle spreads over the posteroinferior endocardial surface of the left ventricle. Peripherally these two fibres are interconnected via the Purkinje fibres. When one of the fascicles is blocked, the impulse is conducted through the other fascicle. As the conduction is very rapid through the fascicles, the fascicular block does not prolong the QRS duration.

Left Anterior Fascicular Block

Left anterior fascicular block is also called left anterior hemiblock (LAHB). LAHB is more common than the block of the posterior fascicle as a single artery supplies the anterior fascicle and it is long and thin, whereas the posterior fascicle has dual blood supply and it is short and thick.

The impulse is not able to pass via the anterior fascicle, so it passes via the posterior fascicle of the left bundle and then the anterior fascicle is activated by the Purkinje fibres distal to the site of the block. The various causes of LAHB are summarized in Box 6.7. The ECG manifestations of LAHB are the following:

1. The QRS axis is deviated to left. The QRS axis lies between −30° and −90°.
2. The normal q wave in leads I and aVL are accentuated.
3. The QRS duration is not prolonged. It is less than 0.12 s.
4. There is a tall R wave in lead I after the prominent q wave.

Box 6.7 Causes of Left Anterior Hemiblock

- Coronary artery disease
- Left ventricular hypertrophy
- Hypertension
- Cardiomyopathy
- Aortic stenosis

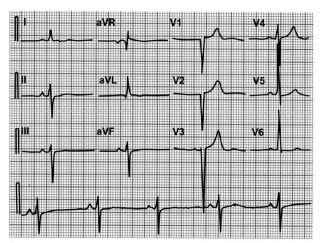

Fig. 6.11   Left anterior hemiblock. This electrocardiogram is taken from a 60-year-old female patient suffering from hypertension for 25 years. Note the deep S waves in leads II and III and the depth of S wave in lead III is more than that of lead II. There is left axis deviation. One must look for these two important features in the beginning.

5. There are deep S waves in leads II and III. The depth of S wave in lead III is more than the depth of S wave in lead II (Fig. 6.11).
6. Prominent initial r waves in leads II, III, and aVF.
7. The normally present small q waves in leads V5 and V6 tend to disappear.
8. The R wave height tends to diminish in leads V5 and V6.
9. The S wave in leads V5 and V6 becomes prominent and there may be terminal slurring.

Left Posterior Fascicular Block

Left posterior fascicular block is also called left posterior hemi-block. It is not very common. It is due to the lesion in the posterior fascicle of the left bundle. Here the impulse is blocked at the left fascicle, and hence, the impulse travels via the anterior fascicle and then via the interconnected Purkinje fibres the impulse travels via the posterior fascicle distal to the block. The ECG manifestations are the following:

1. The QRS axis is deviated to right. It is located between +90° and +120° or +140°.
2. There is prominent S wave in leads I and aVL.

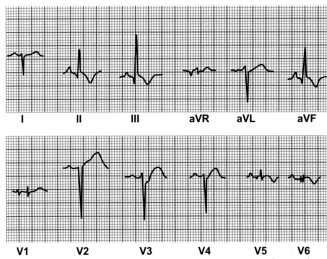

Fig. 6.12 Left posterior fascicular block. It is always important to rule out right ventricular hypertrophy. This patient had come with chest pain and the chest leads show features of anterior wall myocardial infarction.

3. There are prominent R waves in leads II, III, and aVF. The R wave in lead III is the tallest among them (Fig. 6.12).
4. There is a small but prominent q wave in leads II, III, and aVF.
5. There is a small but prominent r wave in lead I.
6. The T wave may be inverted in leads II, III, and aVF.

Left posterior hemiblock is diagnosed only if there is evidence to rule out the possibility of right ventricular hypertrophy and myocardial infarction.

Bilateral Bundle Branch Block

Bilateral bundle branch block is also called bifascicular block. There is block in conduction in both the right and the left bundle. The different types of bilateral bundle branch block are the following:

1. RBBB with LAHB: There is RBBB pattern in chest leads and left axis deviation in standard leads (Fig. 6.13a, b).
2. RBBB with LPHB: It is a very rare combination and the initial 0.08 s determines the axis and the divisional block.
3. RBBB or LBBB with prolonged AV conduction: ECG will reveal RBBB or LBBB with prolonged P–R interval (>0.2 s).

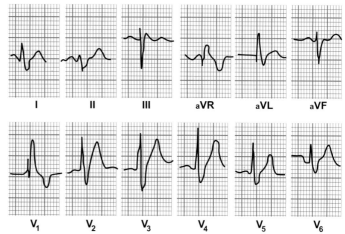

Fig. 6.13a   Right bundle branch block with left anterior hemiblock.

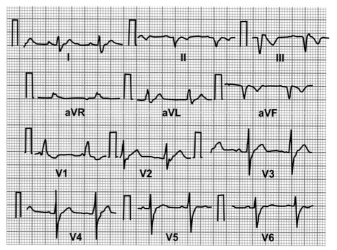

Fig. 6.13b   Right bundle branch block with left anterior hemiblock. Note the broad QRS complex in lead V1 with S–T segment, T wave change. There are also deep S waves in leads II and III and the depth of S wave in lead III is more than that of lead II. Therefore, this is a bifascicular block.

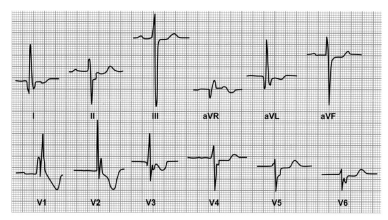

Fig. 6.14 Trifascicular block. There is right bundle branch block with left anterior hemiblock with prolonged P–R interval.

Trifascicular Block

Trifascicular block usually presents as RBBB with LAHB with prolonged P–R interval (first-degree AV block; Fig. 6.14).

BIBLIOGRAPHY

1. Arslan U, Balcioglu S, Tavil Y, et al. Clinical importance of right bundle branch block in the setting of acute anterior myocardial infarction. *J Electrocardiol* 2007; 40(4), S56–S57.
2. Bhargava K, Shrivastava S, Singh B, et al. AV block. Which type and where? *J Electrocardiol* 2007; 40(4), 358–359.
3. Da Costa D, Brady WJ and Edhouse J. Bradycardias and atrioventricular conduction block. *BMJ* 2002; 324(7336), 535–538.
4. Dizadji H, Tahmooressi P and Cernock WF. Etiology of left bundle branch block. Hemodynamic and angiographic studies. *J Electrocardiol* 1974; 7(3), 221–226.
5. Gold FL and From AH. Alternating bundle branch block. *J Electrocardiol* 1980; 13(4), 405–407.
6. Greenwood RJ and Finkelstein D. *Sinoatrial Heart Block*. Charles C. Thomas: Springfield, IL, 1964.

7. Katoh T, Kinoshita S, Tsujimura Y, et al. Repetitive super-normal conduction in the right bundle branch in high degree bilateral bundle branch block. *J Electrocardiol* 2001; 34(2), 179–182.

8. Katoh T, Kinoshita S, Ueji I, et al. Apparent bradycardia-dependent advanced second-degree atrioventricular block. *J Electrocardiol* 2002; 35(2), 153–158.

9. Kupfer JM and Kligfield P. A generalized description of Wenckebach behavior with analysis of determinants of ventricular cycle-length variation during ambulatory electrocardiography. *Am J Cardiol* 1991; 67, 981–986.

10. Ortega-Carnicer J, Gómez-Grande ML and Ambrós A. Right bundle branch block-induced Q waves simulating anterior myocardial infarction extension. *J Electrocardiol* 2000; 33(4), 387–391.

11. Schamroth L and Dove E. The Wenckebach phenomenon in sino-atrial block. *Br Heart J* 1966; 28, 350–358.

12. Smithen CS, Bennett D, Hudson RE, et al. Trifascicular block—an electrocardiographic, hemodynamic and pathological correlation. *J Electrocardiol* 1971; 4(2), 145–152.

13. Wallace AW and Katz LN. Sino-auricular block. *Am Heart J* 1930; 6, 478–482.

CHAPTER 7

Myocardial Ischaemia and Infarction

Chapter Outline

INTRODUCTION

Two most important manifestations of coronary artery disease are myocardial ischaemia and myocardial infarction, and electrocardiogram (ECG) is one of the most important investigations for their evaluation. It is most important for any physician to understand the ECG changes of these conditions, as they are one of the most common emergencies that one has to face every day.

MYOCARDIAL ISCHAEMIA (CORONARY INSUFFICIENCY)

Myocardial ischaemia occurs when adequate blood supply is not available to the myocardium to meet its requirement. Atherosclerosis is the commonest cause of myocardial ischaemia. However, in other conditions such as severe left ventricular hypertrophy (LVH) (aortic stenosis) where the coronary artery is normal, there may be relative ischaemia and angina pectoris. The various causes of myocardial ischaemia are mentioned in Box 7.1.

The ECG changes are mainly seen in S–T segment and T wave in myocardial ischaemia. The changes are, however, not specific of myocardial ischaemia because they can be seen in other conditions such as LVH, pericarditis, myocarditis; hence, the findings should always be correlated with the clinical findings. The diagnosis of myocardial ischaemia should never be made on the basis of ECG results alone.

ECG Features of Myocardial Ischaemia

1. Abnormality of S–T segment
2. Abnormality of T wave
3. Abnormality of U wave

Box 7.1   Causes of Myocardial Ischaemia

- Atherosclerosis
- Severe aortic stenosis
- Polycythaemia
- Anaemia
- Thyroid disorders
- Syphylitic aortitis

S–T SEGMENT ABNORMALITIES

Analysis of S–T segment change is the most important aspect in the diagnosis of myocardial ischaemia. S–T segment change is the commonest electrocardiographic change seen in this condition. This is basically an abnormality of repolarization. S–T segment abnormality may be of two types:

1. S–T segment depression
2. S–T segment elevation

S–T Segment Depression

S–T segment depression is due to the injury of subendocardial area of the left ventricle. Consequently, the S–T segment vector is directed opposite to the surface of the ventricle, i.e., towards the cavity and, therefore, the leads overlying the area will record S–T segment depression. It is recorded best in leads V5 and V6.

S–T segment depression is usually transient and seen during a period of angina but sometimes it may be a permanent feature also. The more the depression, the worse is the prognosis. Sometimes S–T segment depression may not be associated with angina the so-called silent ischaemia. S–T segment depression may be of three types:

1. Horizontal S–T segment depression
2. Up sloping S–T segment depression
3. Down sloping S–T segment depression

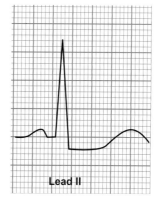

Horizontal S–T Segment Depression

The S–T segment is depressed and leaves the baseline after the QRS complex and merges with the proximal limb of T wave. The horizontality implies the depression of both the proximal and distal part of S–T segment (Fig. 7.1). Almost no part of the S–T segment is isoelectric.

Fig. 7.1 Horizontal S–T segment depression. Note that both the proximal and distal part of the S–T segment is depressed below the baseline.

Up Sloping S–T Segment Depression

Here, only the proximal part of the S–T segment (near its junction with QRS

complex) is depressed. It does not always reflect myocardial ischaemia. It may be seen in sinus tachycardia (Fig. 7.2).

Down Sloping S–T Segment Depression

In this type of S–T segment depression, both the proximal and distal parts of S–T segment are depressed and depression in distal part
is more than that of proximal part (see Fig. 7.3). It reflects severe
coronary insufficiency (see also Fig. 7.4).

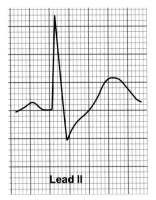

Fig. 7.2 Up sloping S–T segment
depression. Note that the proximal part
of the S–T segment is depressed but
the distal part is not depressed and it is
approaching the baseline.

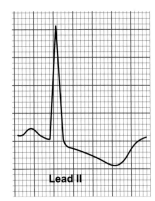

Fig. 7.3 Down sloping S–T segment
depression. Note that the proximal part of
the S–T segment is depressed and the distal
part is also depressed, and the distal part is
more depressed than the proximal part.

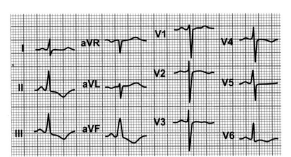

Fig. 7.4 Inferior and anterior wall myocardial ischaemia. This electrocardiogram (ECG)
is recorded from a 65-year-old man who presented with history of severe chest pain with
sweating, palpitation, and dyspnoea. ECG shows down sloping S–T segment depression
in leads II, III, and aVF. Note the inversion of T waves in leads V2, V4, and V6. In the rest of
chest leads, the T waves are flattened. Results from coronary angiography revealed more
than 90% block in left anterior descending coronary artery and 75% block in right coronary artery. He underwent coronary bypass surgery for revascularization.

S–T Segment Elevation

S–T segment elevation is not a common finding in myocardial ischaemia, rather it points more towards myocardial infarction. It represents transmural ischaemia. S–T segment elevation occurs in Prinzmetal's angina (coronary vasospasm). The S–T segment elevation is associated with a tall and widened T wave and the S–T segment tends to be concave upwards (Fig. 7.5). When chest pain subsides, the S–T segment usually becomes isoelectric. It is a feature of transmural epicardial injury. Here the vector is directed towards the surface of injury and, therefore, the overlying leads record S–T segment elevation. Various ECG features of Prinzmetal's angina are mentioned in Box 7.2.

The various causes of S–T segment changes are summarized in Box 7.3.

T WAVE ABNORMALITIES

T wave is inverted in myocardial ischaemia. The inverted T wave has symmetrical limbs with a narrow, pointed nadir (arrowhead appearance). Inverted T waves sometimes become upright during coronary insufficiency. Even though the ECG will appear normal, it is indicative

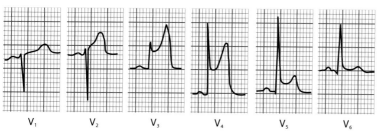

V_1 V_2 V_3 V_4 V_5 V_6

Fig. 7.5 Prinzmetal's angina. This electrocardiogram (ECG) is recorded from a 39-year-old man suffering from severe chest pain. ECG revealed tall R waves in leads V4 and V5 along with tall T waves with slope elevation in leads V2–V5. Coronary angiography did not reveal any gross abnormality. It was due to coronary artery spasm.

Box 7.2 Electrocardiogram Features of Prinzmetal's Angina

- S–T segment elevation
- Increase in amplitude of R wave
- Decrease in depth of S wave
- Inversion of U wave
- Ventricular extrasystoles
- Atrioventricular block

Box 7.3   Changes in S–T Segment

S–T Segment Elevation
- Acute myocardial infarction (transmural)
- Ventricular aneurysm
- Pericarditis
- Prinzmetal's angina
- Early repolarization syndrome
- Cerebrovascular accident

S–T Segment Depression
- Myocardial ischaemia
- Subendocardial infarction
- Digitalis effect
- Digitalis toxicity
- Myocarditis
- Cardiomyopathy
- Cerebrovascular accident

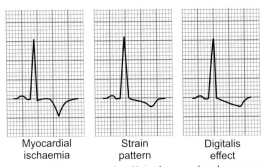

| Myocardial | Strain | Digitalis |
| ischaemia | pattern | effect |

Fig. 7.6   Three types of T wave inversion. Note the arrowhead appearance in myocardial ischaemia, the asymmetry of T wave in strain pattern, and the reverse check sign in digitalis effect.

of further coronary insufficiency. In strain pattern (LVH), the T wave is inverted but asymmetric. In digitalis effect, the T wave is inverted but asymmetrical and the nadir is blunted (Fig. 7.6).

U WAVE ABNORMALITIES

U waves are inverted in myocardial ischaemia. Inversion of U wave is also seen in hypertensive heart disease. The various ECG changes of myocardial ischaemia are summarized in Box 7.4.

Box 7.4   Electrocardiogram Features of Myocardial Ischaemia

- S–T segment depression (down sloping or horizontal)
- S–T segment elevation (Prinzmetal's angina)
- T wave inversion
- Inversion of U wave

MYOCARDIAL INFARCTION

Myocardial infarction occurs due to interruption of blood supply to a part of myocardium that results in necrosis of myocardium. The commonest cause is complete occlusion of coronary artery due to rupture of an atherosclerotic plaque (Fig. 7.7a). The same process that produces myocardial ischaemia can produce myocardial infarction. However, the myocardium is sometimes spared if there is a good collateral circulation. In almost all the cases, there is infarction of the left ventricle and the right ventricle is involved in association with left ventricle.

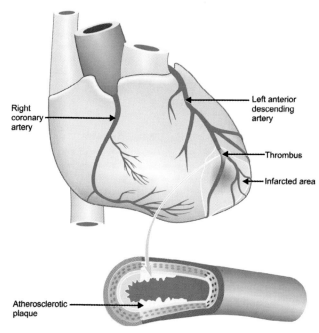

Fig. 7.7a   Myocardial infarction.

ECG is the most valuable and initial investigation in the diagnosis of myocardial infarction. Similar ECG changes may be seen in other conditions such as pericarditis, ventricular aneurysm and hence, in all the cases history of the patient should be considered before interpreting ECG results. It must be kept in mind that sometimes myocardial infarction may not be associated with all the ECG changes. A single ECG recorded may not reveal the changes of infarction but serial ECG tracings are often required to arrive at the correct diagnosis.

Currently it has been observed that previously used terms such as transmural and subendocardial infarction are no longer tenable because they do not match with the pathological findings at autopsy. Now, the present terminology is based on the presence or absence of Q waves. If the Q waves are present in ECG it is called *Q wave myocardial infarction* and if they are absent it is called *non-Q myocardial infarction*.

In a fully evolved case of infarction there is a central zone of necrosis (Fig. 7.7b, c). This zone is surrounded by a zone of injury, which in turn is surrounded by a zone of ischaemia.

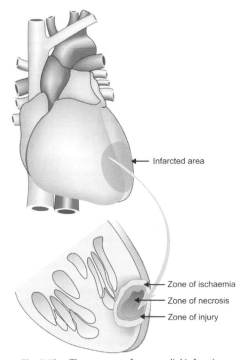

Fig. 7.7b   Three zones of myocardial infarction.

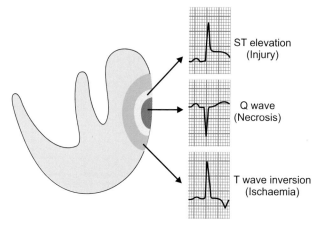

Fig. 7.7c   Electrocardiogram manifestation of three zones of myocardial infarction.

Myocardial Necrosis

Myocardial necrosis is manifested in ECG by Q waves and loss of amplitude of R waves. It is represented by the QS complex. It is a totally negative complex. The necrosed myocardium cannot be depolarized and, therefore, is electrically inert and produces an electrical window. The lead over the window records the electrical activity of the healthy myocardium through the window. Because the electrical wavefront is moving away from the lead (interventricular septum), it will record a negative deflection, which is the Q wave (Fig. 7.8). After this, the electrode will record the wavefront of depolarization of the distant free wall which is also moving away from the electrode and, therefore, another negative deflection will be recorded. The QRS vector is thus directed completely away from the infarcted myocardium.

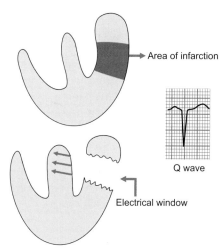

Fig. 7.8   Genesis of 'Q' wave.

The pathological Q wave is more than 0.04 s in duration and more than 4 mm in depth or more than 25% deep than the height of R wave (Fig. 7.9). In lead III and sometimes in lead aVL, Q waves are seen normally which are 0.04 s in duration and the Q-to-R ratio is greater than 25%. Therefore, diagnosis of infarction should not be made on the basis of lead III alone.

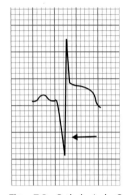

Fig. 7.9 Pathological Q wave. Note the depth and width of the Q wave (arrow).

Myocardial Injury

Myocardial injury is manifested in ECG by S–T segment elevation. This is often the first ECG change of myocardial infarction. The S–T segment is elevated and is convex or curved upwards. The lead oriented to the injured epicardial surface records S–T segment elevation and the lead oriented to the uninjured surface records S–T segment depression (cavity lead aVR). S–T segment elevation is commonly recorded because most of the infarctions are transmural infarctions.

Myocardial Ischaemia

Myocardial ischaemia is reflected electrocardiographically by inverted, symmetrical, and pointed T waves. These inverted T waves are also increased in amplitude. The 'coronary T' or 'Pardee T' means inverted T wave with isoelectric S–T segment, which has upward convexity. The 'cove plane T' means T wave inversion in a lead with S–T segment elevation with convexity upwards. However, in the very early phase of infarction often the T wave becomes very tall and upright. After this the T wave inversion takes place. Sometimes, the T wave inversion persists for the rest of the patient's life, but most of the times it becomes normal.

An electrode oriented towards the infarcted myocardium will record all the three changes of myocardial infarction.

Evolution of Myocardial Infarction

The evolution of infarction occurs through three phases, which can be recorded by ECG. They are:

1. The hyperacute phase
2. Fully evolved phase
3. Chronic stable phase

Hyperacute Phase of Infarction

Hyperacute phase occurs in the first few hours after onset of myocardial infarction. It occurs before the fully evolved phase and is a critical phase in the evolution of infarction. During this phase, the patient has a chance of developing life threatening ventricular fibrillation. This stage is also important because thrombolytic therapy during this phase is extremely beneficial for the patient. The ECG manifestations are the following:

1. Tall R waves
2. Increased ventricular activation time
3. Slope elevation of S–T segment
4. Tall and wide T waves (Fig. 7.10)

Fully Evolved Phase

In fully evolved phase of myocardial infarction Q waves, S–T segment elevation and T wave inversion are recorded. Often, the hyperacute phase is not observed, because the patient may visit the hospital late and the ECG taken at that time reflects the fully evolved phase of myocardial infarction.

Chronic Stable Phase

After the fully evolved phase, there is gradual resolution of the ECG changes. At first, the S–T segment becomes isoelectric. After that the

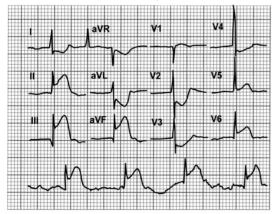

Fig. 7.10 Hyperacute inferior wall myocardial infarction. Hyperacute infarction is indicated by tall R waves with slope elevation of T waves in leads II, III, and aVF. There is reciprocal depression of S–T segment in leads I, aVL, and V2–V4. The S–T segment in leads V5 and V6 is also elevated. This patient is also developing lateral wall infarction.

T waves become upright. The Q waves usually persist and remain as marker of old myocardial infarction. After 1 year, about 30% of ECGs are no longer diagnostic of myocardial infarction. The various phases of evolution are shown in Fig. 7.11.

Subendocardial Infarction

Subendocardial infarction is manifested electrocardiographically by S–T segment depression and T wave inversion. These abnormalities persist for several days. Q waves are absent in subendocardial infarction (Fig. 7.12). This is called non-Q myocardial infarction now. The S–T segment depression persists for several days without

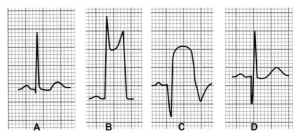

Fig. 7.11   Various phases of evolution of myocardial infarction. (A) Normal PQRST complex. (B) Hyperacute phase. (C) Fully evolved phase. (D) Chronic stable phase.

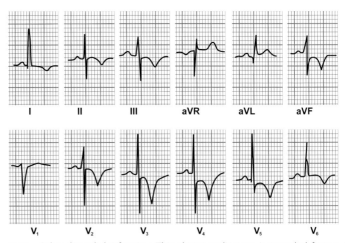

Fig. 7.12   Subendocardial infarction. This electrocardiogram is recorded from a 72-year-old man suffering from severe chest pain with left ventricular failure. Note the deep and symmetrical T wave inversion in leads V2–V5. The T waves are also inverted in leads II, III, and aVF. During the hospital stay there was never any S–T segment elevation.

any appearance of Q waves. However, during this time the serum cardiac markers (enzymes) are elevated.

Localization of Myocardial Infarction

Myocardial infarction involves mainly the left ventricle. Sometimes the right ventricle and the atria are also involved. The coronary artery developing atherosclerotic blockage or undergoing coronary spasm can be guessed by the leads showing S–T, T changes as shown in Box 7.5.

Left Ventricular Infarction

Left ventricle is infarcted in almost all the patients suffering from myocardial infarction. The following areas of left ventricle may be infarcted

1. Anterior wall
2. Inferior wall
3. Posterior wall (Fig. 7.13)

Box 7.5 Prediction of Blockage of Coronary Artery	
Leads showing S–T, T change	**Coronary artery blocked**
• Leads V1–V4	Left anterior descending coronary artery
• Leads I, aVL, V5, and V6	Left circumflex coronary artery
• Leads II, III, and aVF	Right coronary artery

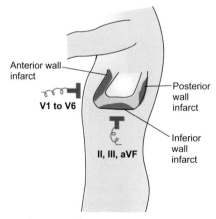

Fig. 7.13   Illustration of anterior, inferior, and posterior wall myocardial infarction.

Anterior Wall Myocardial Infarction

The anterior wall infarction may be arbitrarily subdivided into the following types.

1. Extensive anterior wall infarction: The changes are located in leads I, aVL, and V1–V6 (Figs. 7.14 and 7.15).
2. Anteroseptal infarction: The changes are located in leads V1–V4.
3. Anterolateral infarction: The changes are located in leads I, aVL, V5, and V6.
4. Apical infarction: The changes are located in leads V5 and V6 (Fig. 7.16).

Inferior Wall Myocardial Infarction

The changes of inferior wall myocardial infarction are located in leads II, III, and aVF (Fig. 7.17a–c). A small q wave may be normally present in lead III that usually disappears on deep inspiration. So, lead III should be routinely recorded in deep inspiration. Sinus bradycardia is often seen in inferior wall infarction. S–T segment

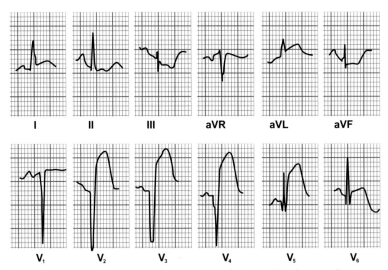

Fig. 7.14 Extensive anterior wall myocardial infarction. This electrocardiogram is recorded from a 55-year-old woman suffering from severe chest pain with left ventricular failure. She was also suffering from diabetes mellitus that was not under control. Note the S–T segment elevation with convexity upwards in leads V2–V6. Note that there is a rising trend of S–T segment in leads I and aVL.

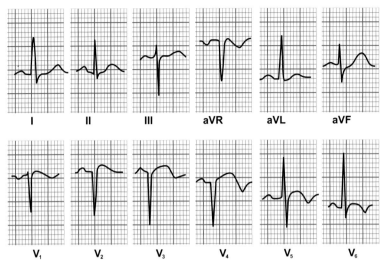

I   II   III   aVR   aVL   aVF

V₁   V₂   V₃   V₄   V₅   V₆

Fig. 7.15 Anterior wall myocardial infarction. This electrocardiogram is recorded from a 67-year-old man suffering from severe chest pain with vomiting, sweating, and left ventricular failure. He was also suffering from diabetes mellitus and hypercholesterolaemia. Note the S–T segment elevation with convexity upwards in leads V2–V6. Note that there is also a rising trend of S–T segment in lead V1.

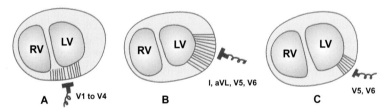

Fig. 7.16 Illustration of infarction of various walls of left ventricle. (A) Anteroseptal infarction. (B) Anterolateral infarction. (C) Apical infarction.

elevation and T wave inversion in leads II, III, and aVF may produce reciprocal changes in the form of S–T segment depression and tall T waves in leads I, aVL, and V1–V6.

Posterior Wall Myocardial Infarction

Posterior wall infarction rarely occurs alone. It is usually associated with inferior wall infarction. None of the leads of the conventional 12 lead ECG is directly oriented towards the posterior wall of the heart. Therefore, the leads opposite to the posterior wall, i.e., anterior wall will record the inverse or the mirror image changes.

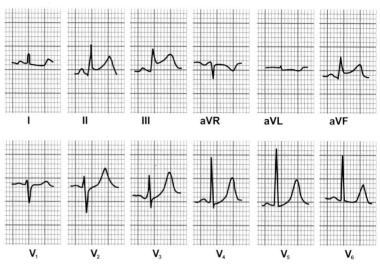

Fig. 7.17a Hyperacute inferior wall myocardial infarction. This electrocardiogram (ECG) is recorded from a 73-year-old man suffering from severe chest pain with vomiting, sweating, and left ventricular failure. He was also suffering from diabetes mellitus. Note the slope elevation of S–T segment in leads II, III, and aVF. This is a very early stage of infarction.

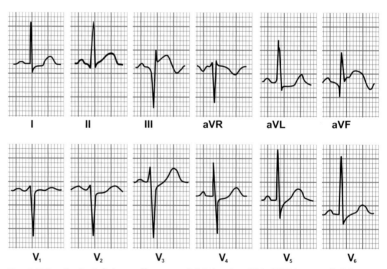

Fig. 7.17b Acute inferior wall myocardial infarction. This ECG is recorded from a 74-year-old man suffering from severe chest pain with vomiting, sweating, and palpitation. He was also suffering from diabetes mellitus and hypertriglyceridaemia. Note the S–T segment elevation with convexity upwards in leads II, III, and aVF.

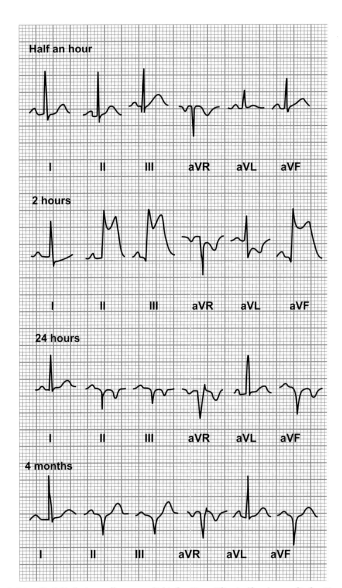

Fig. 7.17c Serial inferior wall myocardial infarction. After half an hour of infarction S–T segment is slightly elevated. After 2 hours the hyperacute phase is recorded. After 24 hours the Q waves are recorded in lead III along with T wave inversion. After 4 months, only the Q waves are persisting. The T waves are upright.

Thus, the changes are recorded in leads V1–V3, especially lead V2 (Fig. 7.18). The changes in lead V2 are:

1. Tall and slightly wide R wave (mirror image of QS complex).
2. Depressed and concave upwards S–T segment (mirror image of convex upwards S–T segment elevation).
3. Upright, tall, and wide T wave (mirror image of inverted T wave).

Right Ventricular Infarction

Isolated right ventricular infarction is very rare. It is usually associated with inferior wall infarction. The various probable causes of less incidence of right ventricular infarction are thin wall of right ventricle, rich collateral circulation, and low pressure in right ventricle. Right ventricular infarction should be suspected in the presence of inferior wall infarction if the following changes are recorded:

1. S–T segment elevation in leads V1 and V4R (Fig. 7.19).
2. S–T segment depression in lead V2 is 50% or less than the magnitude of S–T segment elevation in lead aVF.

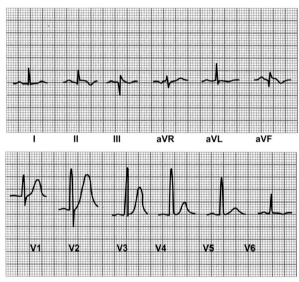

Fig. 7.18   Posterior and inferior wall infarction. This electrocardiogram is recorded from a 72-year-old man suffering from chest pain with vomiting and sweating. Note the tall R and T wave in leads V1 and V2 indicative of posterior wall infarction. There are Q waves with T wave inversion in leads II, III, and aVF, which indicates inferior wall infarction.

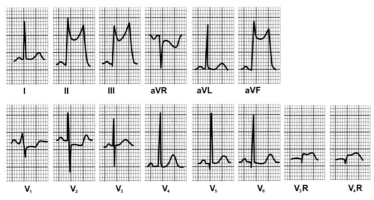

Fig.7.19 Inferior and right ventricular infarction. Note the tall R waves in leads II, III, and aVF with slope elevation of S–T segment indicative of hyperacute inferior wall infarction. There is S–T segment elevation in leads V3R and V4R, which indicates right ventricular infarction.

3. S–T segment elevation in leads V1–V4 but the maximum elevation will be in lead V1 and the elevation decreases from V1 to V4. Q waves will be absent in these leads.

4. S–T segment elevation in lead V1 and S–T segment depression in lead V2.

Myocardial Infarction in the Presence of Left Bundle Branch Block

Myocardial infarction is difficult to diagnose in the presence of left bundle branch block (LBBB). The following features are indicative of infarction in presence of LBBB.

1. Q wave duration of ≥ 0.04 s in leads V5 and V6.
2. Serial S–T segment and T wave changes.
3. Q wave of any magnitude in lead V6.

Myocardial Infarction in the Presence of Right Bundle Branch Block

Anterior wall myocardial infarction in the presence of right bundle branch block (RBBB) will lead to disappearance of the initial r wave of the rSR' complex in leads V1, V2, or V3. There will be a QS complex in these leads. In general, RBBB does not hide the features of myocardial infarction unlike LBBB (see Fig. 7.20).

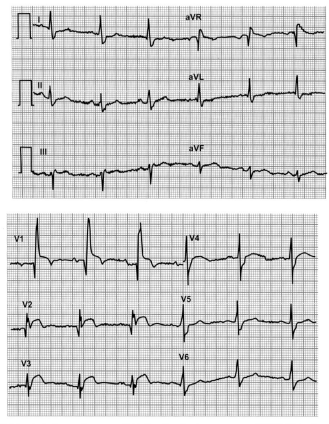

Fig. 7.20 Anterior wall myocardial infarction in the presence of RBBB. This electrocardiogram (ECG) is recorded from a 56-year-old man who was suffering from coronary artery disease. He had RBBB in his earlier ECG tracings taken during his previous admission. He was now admitted with severe chest pain with sweating and vomiting. ECG revealed S–T segment elevation in leads V1–V4, which signifies anteroseptal myocardial infarction.

BIBLIOGRAPHY

1. Barold SS. Diagnosis of inferior myocardial infarction based on the paced QRS complex. *J Electrocardiol* 2007; 40(2), 161–163.

2. Buszman P, Szafranek A, Kalarus Z, et al. Use of changes in ST segment elevation for prediction of infarct artery recanalization in acute myocardial infarction. *Eur Heart J* 1995; 16, 1207–1214.

3. Francis M and William JB. ABC of clinical electrocardiography: Acute myocardial infarction—Part I. *BMJ* 2002; 324, 831–834.

4. Istratoaie O, Mustafa R, Dominic ID, et al. Evolutive features of transmural myocardial infarction with hyperacute T wave in early phases. *J Electrocardiol* 2007; 40(4), S58.

5. June E, William JB and Francis M. ABC of clinical electrocardiography: Acute myocardial infarction—Part II. *BMJ* 2002; 324, 963–966.

6. Karlson BW, Herlitz J, Wiklund O, et al. Early prediction of acute myocardial infarction from clinical history, examination and electrocardiogram in the emergency room. *Am J Cardiol* 1991; 68, 171–175.

7. Kevin C and Francis M. ABC of clinical electrocardiography: Myocardial ischaemia. *BMJ* 2002; 324, 1023–1026.

CHAPTER 8

Cardiac Rhythm Disturbances

Chapter Outline

INTRODUCTION

The normal cardiac rhythm depends on the spontaneous generation of impulse by the sinoatrial (SA) node and its proper conduction through the conducting system of the heart. Disturbance in any of the two (generation or conduction of impulse) will lead to rhythm disturbances. The SA node acts as the pacemaker of the heart as it has the fastest inherent rate of impulse generation (70–80 beats/min). However, there are also several other potential pacemakers of the heart. These are present in atria, atrioventricular (AV) junctional area, bundle branches, Purkinje fibres etc. If SA node fails to generate the impulse, the other structures will take up the pacemaker function. The rates of inherent discharge of these other pacemakers are slow. Thus, the usual rate of discharge of AV node is 60 beats/min, bundle of His is 50 beats/min, and ventricular myocardium is 30–45 beats/min.

AV NODE ELECTROPHYSIOLOGY

AV junction area is made up of the following parts:

1. Area of junction of atria and AV node
2. AV node proper
3. Area of junction of AV node and His bundle

The cells of the AV node proper do not have automaticity and therefore never act as the pacemaker of the heart, but this area has the property of slowing down the conduction that contributes a large part of the P–R interval. The other two areas have the property of automaticity and may act as the pacemaker in pathological conditions.

SINUS RHYTHM

Normal sinus rhythm reflects the normal electrical activity of the heart. The SA node is the pacemaker of the heart and the rate of discharge is governed by the sympathetic and parasympathetic system. The normal sinus rate of discharge is between 60 and 100 beats/min and this is the normal heart rate. Whenever the impulse originates at a normal rate from the SA node it is called sinus rhythm. This is seen in electrocardiogram (ECG) by the normal P wave followed by the normal QRST complexes. The P–R interval and QRS complex are normal (Fig. 8.1a, b).

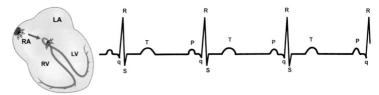

Fig 8.1a   Illustration of genesis of normal sinus rhythm. The impulse originates at SA node at a rate between 60 and 100 beats/min and travels via the normal conducting system to the ventricles.

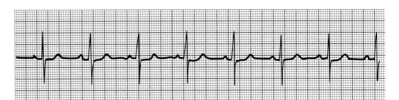

Fig 8.1b   Normal sinus rhythm. The rhythm is regular and the heart rate is 72 beats/min. The P–R interval and QRS duration are normal.

SINUS TACHYCARDIA

Sinus tachycardia is a normal response of the heart to the demand for excess blood flow (e.g., exercise, exertion). When the SA node generates impulse at a rate greater than 100 beats/min, it is called sinus tachycardia. The P, QRS, and T waves are normal but are in rapid succession. In adults, usually, sinus tachycardia does not exceed 160 beats/min. The P–R interval and QRS duration are normal. It is a physiological response to exercise, anxiety etc. It can occur due to fever, thyrotoxicosis, cardiac failure, myocarditis, shock, drugs (e.g., adrenaline, atropine), etc. (Fig. 8.2). If sinus tachycardia does not occur in conditions such as fever, exercise, thyrotoxicosis, then it may be due to underlying SA nodal disease such as sick sinus syndrome.

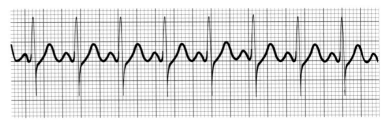

Fig 8.2   Sinus tachycardia. The heart rate is 125 beats/min.

SINUS BRADYCARDIA

Sinus bradycardia is a normal body response to relaxation, sleep etc. When the SA node generates impulse at a rate less than 60 beats/min, it is called sinus bradycardia. The P, QRS, and T waves are normal but are in slow succession. The various causes of sinus tachycardia and sinus bradycardia are summarized in Box 8.1. Sinus bradycardia is a manifestation of SA nodal disease but the common causes such as hypothyroidism, beta-blocker therapy should be ruled out in the beginning (Fig. 8.3).

Box 8.1   Causes of Sinus Tachycardia and Sinus Bradycardia

Sinus Tachycardia
- Exercise, emotion, pain
- Anxiety
- Thyrotoxicosis
- Fever
- Excessive tea and coffee consumption
- Atropine and adrenaline administration
- Heart failure
- Shock
- Hypoxia
- Pulmonary embolism
- Myocardial infarction

Sinus Bradycardia
- Athletes
- Deep sleep
- Beta-blockers
- Raised intracranial tension
- Hypothermia
- Obstructive jaundice
- Diseases of SA node
- Digitalis effect
- Inferior wall myocardial infarction
- Sick sinus syndrome

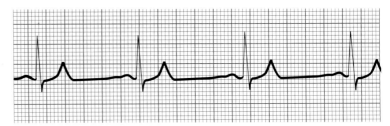

Fig 8.3   Sinus bradycardia. The heart rate is 54 beats/min.

SINUS ARRHYTHMIA

In sinus arrhythmia, the impulse originates at the SA node but in an irregular manner. It is characterized by alternating periods of fast and slow discharge of SA node. This is usually associated with the phases of respiration and, therefore, called respiratory sinus arrhythmia. The slow rate occurs at the end of expiration and the faster rate occurs at the end of inspiration (Fig. 8.4). The heart rate may be normal (60–100 beats/min). It is a normal physiological phenomenon and is prominent in young children. During inspiration there is increased venous return to heart, vagal tone decreases, and heart rate increases. During expiration venous return decreases, vagal tone increases, and heart rate decreases.

The P waves and QRS complexes are normal. The P–R interval and QRS duration are also normal. The difference between the longest and the shortest R–R interval is greater than 0.12 s. It is commonly associated with sinus bradycardia.

ATRIAL ARRHYTHMIAS

Atrial arrhythmias originate from an ectopic focus in the atria. The main feature is the different morphology of the P wave from the sinus P wave as it originates from a different focus. The P wave may

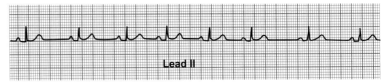

Fig 8.4   Sinus arrhythmia. Note the tachycardia during inspiration and bradycardia during expiration. Also note that every QRS complex is preceded by a P wave and they bear a constant relationship.

be pointed, notched, inverted etc. If the atrial rate is very fast, then P wave may not be visible or it may be superimposed on preceding T wave or there may be saw-tooth appearance or a wavy baseline.

There are mainly five types of atrial rhythm disturbances. They arise from ectopic focus either in atrium or in AV node.

1. Atrial extrasystoles
2. Wandering atrial pacemaker
3. Paroxysmal atrial tachycardia (PAT)
4. Atrial flutter
5. Atrial fibrillation

Atrial Extrasystoles

Atrial extrasystoles are atrial premature beats. The premature atrial contraction is an early (premature in timing) beat that originates from an ectopic atrial focus that discharges before the next sinus beat and thus interrupts the rhythm. They arise from atrial muscle (not from SA node) and the wave front passes in the atria through abnormal pathway resulting in abnormal, bizarre P' wave. The P' wave may be hidden in the preceding T wave resulting in alteration of contour of the T wave. The QRS complex will be normal. The impulse may originate from anywhere in either atrium (Fig. 8.5a, b).

Atrial premature beats are commonly observed in normal persons. They may occur due to emotional disturbance, excess tea, coffee, or tobacco consumption, etc. Almost any type of heart disease can lead to ectopic atrial beats. Digitalis is a known cause of atrial extrasystoles. The various causes of atrial extrasystoles are summarized in Box 8.2. Three or more than three consecutive atrial extrasystoles constitute atrial tachycardia. Frequent multifocal atrial extrasystoles may precipitate atrial fibrillation.

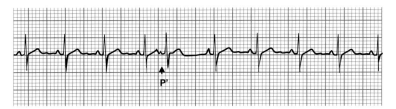

Fig 8.5a   Atrial extrasystoles. The P' wave is shown with an arrow. Note the different configuration from the sinus P waves. Also note the incomplete pause after the atrial extrasystoles.

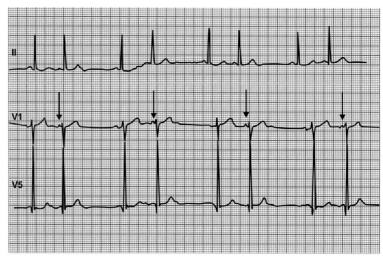

Fig 8.5b Atrial bigeminy. The P' waves are shown with an arrow. The extrasystoles are occurring after every sinus beat. Note their different configuration from the sinus P waves. Also note the incomplete pause after the atrial extrasystoles.

Box.8.2.   Causes of Atrial Extrasystoles

- Normal phenomenon
- Excessive tea, coffee, and tobacco consumption
- Coronary, thyrotoxic, rheumatic, hypertensive heart disease
- Drugs—Digitalis, adrenaline, thyroxin
- Pulmonary embolism
- Hypokalaemia, hypomagnesaemia

The characteristics of atrial extrasystoles are the following:

1. The P' wave occurs earlier than the anticipated P wave. It may be upright, biphasic, inverted, flattened, notched, pointed, or may be lost in preceding T wave.
2. The QRS complex following the P' wave is usually normal.
3. The compensatory pause following the atrial extrasystole is incomplete. This means that the total duration of the pre- and post-extrasystolic R–R interval is less than twice the normal R–R interval.
4. The P'–R interval may be normal, short, or prolonged.

Treatment of Atrial Extrasystoles

Mostly the patients are asymptomatic and treatment is not required but factors that trigger extrasystoles such as alcohol, tea, coffee, adrenergic stimulants should be avoided. Sometimes mild sedatives or beta-blockers are required.

Wandering Atrial Pacemaker

Wandering pacemaker, as the name suggests is characterized by the origin of impulses from the SA node as well as from various other foci located in various parts of atria and AV junction. This leads to various types of P' waves with variation in rhythm and changing P'–R intervals. At least three different types of P wave morphologies must be identified before making a diagnosis (Fig. 8.6). This arrhythmia can occur in normal persons and in various types of heart diseases such as acute rheumatic fever, myocarditis, digitalis toxicity, sick sinus syndrome. The main ECG features are:

1. P waves are of different morphology
2. P–P and R–R intervals may vary
3. QRS duration is normal
4. Heart rate is normal or there may be bradycardia
5. P–R interval is usually normal but may vary

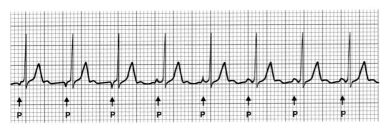

Fig 8.6   Wandering atrial pacemaker. Note the different morphologies of P waves.

Paroxysmal Atrial Tachycardia

Paroxysmal atrial tachycardia is manifested electrocardiographically by three or more than three atrial extrasystoles at a regular rate of 160–230 beats/min. It is also known as paroxysmal supraventricular tachycardia (PSVT). The tachycardia occurs in bursts, i.e., it starts abruptly and ends abruptly. It is associated with a normal or nearly normal QRS complex. The QRS complex may be widened if there is intraventricular conduction defect. The P' wave is difficult to identify as it is merged with the T wave of the

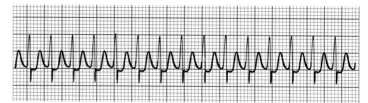

Fig 8.7 Paroxysmal atrial tachycardia. Note the regular and rapid ventricular rate with the absence of P wave and the S–T segment depression.

preceding complex. If the P' waves are seen, they may be flattened, notched, pointed, or biphasic. P–R interval is usually not measurable (Fig. 8.7).

PAT is often seen in persons in whom there is no evidence of heart disease. It is commonly associated with Wolff–Parkinson–White (WPW) syndrome. It occurs more commonly in patients with an accessory conduction pathway, coronary artery disease, mitral valve prolapse, digitalis toxicity etc. PAT may last for a few seconds or may last for a few days. Patients usually complain of palpitation and they must be first reassured that they are not suffering from a catastrophic heart disease.

Treatment

Vagal manoeuvre such as carotid massage and valsalva manoeuvre terminates tachycardia in majority of the patients. Intravenous adenosine is the drug of choice for treatment. Six to twelve milligram is given IV to terminate the arrhythmia. IV verapamil is also very effective. Digitalis is contraindicated in acute management. If these measures fail, then electrical cardioversion (25–50 Ws) is done especially in the presence of hypotension or ischaemia. The bypass tract should be detected and treated by radiofrequency catheter ablation.

Atrial Flutter

Atrial flutter originates from an ectopic atrial focus that discharges in a regular and rapid rate of 230–350 beats/min. The P' waves of atrial flutter produce a 'saw tooth' appearance of the base line (Fig. 8.8). The flutter wave (F wave) is best seen in leads II and VI. The flutter wave affects the baseline in such a way that there is no isoelectric line and T wave is partially or completely obscured by flutter waves. AV block of varying degrees (2:1, 3:1, or 4:1) exist and the

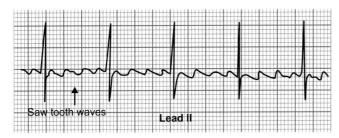

Fig 8.8: Atrial flutter with 4:1 conduction. Note the saw-tooth waves (arrow).

ventricular rate is slower than the atrial rate. The QRS complexes are normal unless there is a bundle branch block or aberrant ventricular conduction. If the conduction ratio remains constant (e.g., 4:1), then ventricular rhythm will be regular, and if, the conduction ratio varies (e.g., from 2:1 to 3:1 or 4:1) then ventricular rhythm will be irregular. When ventricular rate is less than 100 beats/min then atrial flutter is termed 'controlled' and when the ventricular rate is more than 100 beats/min then it is called 'uncontrolled.'

Atrial flutter may be seen in normal individuals but usually, it is seen in patients suffering from coronary artery disease, rheumatic heart disease, thyrotoxicosis, pulmonary embolism etc. Often flutter coexists with atrial fibrillation, in which case it is called flutter-fibrillation.

Treatment

Approximately 25–50 Ws electrical cardioversion is the main treatment under mild sedation. Beta-blocker and calcium channel blocker are used to reduce ventricular rate. Digitalis is better avoided as it may convert flutter into atrial fibrillation. After slowing ventricular rate amiodarone or ibutilide (new anti-arrhythmic drug) may be used to convert into sinus rhythm. Radiofrequency catheter ablation may be used where re-entry is the cause of atrial flutter.

Atrial Fibrillation

Atrial fibrillation occurs when multiple ectopic foci in atria (or via re-entry mechanism) discharges at a rate between 400 and 600 beats/min. Atrial fibrillation is an absolutely irregular atrial rhythm. It is commonly observed in coronary artery disease, rheumatic heart disease, thyrotoxicosis, etc. It may also be seen in normal persons. Paroxysm of atrial fibrillation is seen in thyrotoxicosis and WPW syndrome. Sometimes it is not associated with any disease which is called lone atrial fibrillation. The various causes of atrial fibrillation are summarized in Box 8.3.

Patients usually suffer from palpitation and sometimes they may also be asymptomatic. However, continuous atrial fibrillation may lead to thrombus formation in the atrium, which may further lead to embolism. Besides this, long-standing atrial fibrillation may lead to hypertrophy of heart. So, always an attempt should be made to convert them into sinus rhythm. The prognosis lies in the underlying cardiac disease.

In atrial fibrillation, the depolarization and repolarization of the atria is disorganized and chaotic and hence at a given time, part of atria is in excited state and part of it is in recovery state. These numerous impulses reach the AV node at irregular intervals at a very high frequency, which overwhelms the AV node. AV node conducts some of these impulses and block most of them during its refractory state. These in turn excite the ventricles irregularly at a fairly rapid rate. This leads to irregular atrial and ventricular rhythm.

Box 8.3   Causes of Atrial Fibrillation

- Rheumatic fever
- Mitral stenosis
- Thyrotoxicosis
- Drugs—adrenaline, digitalis
- Cor pulmonale
- Excessive consumption of tea, coffee, alcohol
- Constrictive pericarditis
- Lone atrial fibrillation
- Acute myocardial infarction
- Sick sinus syndrome
- Cardiac surgery
- Pulmonary embolism
- Paroxysmal atrial fibrillation in young person after consumption of alcohol—'Holiday Heart Syndrome'
- Cardiomyopathy
- Hypertensive heart disease

Atrial fibrillation is diagnosed by the following features:

1. Irregularly irregular ventricular rhythm with normal QRS complexes. The ventricular rate is usually 120–160 beats/min. This leads to varying R–R interval. Ventricular rate may be regular because of digitalis toxicity.
2. The P waves are replaced by fibrillatory waves (f waves) resulting in a wavy baseline. Atrial rate is 350–400 beats/min. There is no identifiable P wave (Fig. 8.9a, b).

Treatment

In presence of severe cardiovascular compromise, electrical cardioversion (100 Ws) is the main treatment. Beta-blocker or calcium channel blocker may achieve reduction of ventricular rate by increasing the AV node refractory period. Rapid digitalization is an alternative. For chronic therapy digitalis, beta-blocker or calcium channel blockers are used to reduce the ventricular rate. In some cases, cardioversion (with prior anticoagulation) may be attempted to convert into sinus rhythm. Treatment of underlying causes such as thyrotoxicosis, pericarditis, congestive heart failure (CHF) should be done.

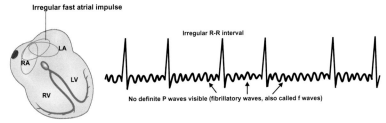

Fig 8.9a   Illustration of genesis of atrial fibrillation.

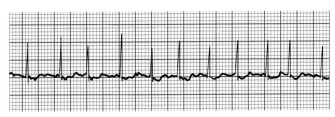

Fig 8.9b   Atrial fibrillation. Note the irregularly irregular R–R interval. The P waves are replaced by fibrillatory waves (wavy baseline).

AV JUNCTIONAL/NODAL RHYTHM

An impulse may originate from the AV junction instead of the SA node and is called AV junctional/nodal rhythm. It must be kept in mind that the rhythm does not originate from the AV node because it has no property of generation of impulse. The impulse may be conducted to the atria and the ventricles. The impulse may be conducted to the ventricles only and the retrograde conduction to the atria may be blocked.

When the impulse is conducted to both the atria and the ventricles, then the ventricular activation proceeds along the normal pathway resulting in normal QRS complex. The conduction to the atria occurs in a retrograde manner, i.e., the direction of depolarization is reversed resulting in inverted P waves in leads II, III, and aVF and upright in lead aVR. This P wave may precede or follow or may be hidden in the QRS complex. This depends on the relative velocity of the anterograde and retrograde conduction. This nodal rhythm may be in the form of AV nodal extrasystole, AV nodal escape beat, paroxysmal AV nodal tachycardia, or idionodal tachycardia. In all these arrhythmias, the features are similar to that described in atrial arrhythmias except that the P waves will be inverted and may appear before, after or hidden in QRS complex.

Premature Junctional Complex

The ECG features of premature junctional complex is similar to that of premature atrial complex except that the P' wave will be inverted. It may appear before, after, or hidden in the QRS complex (Fig. 8.10).

Junctional Rhythm

Junctional rhythm arises from AV junction at a rate between 40 and 60 beats/min. This rhythm occurs when the discharge rate

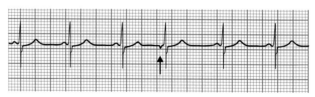

Fig 8.10   Premature junctional complex. Note the inverted P' wave of fourth complex which is followed by a pause.

of SA node falls and the AV junction takes over as the dominant pacemaker (Fig. 8.11). The ECG features are:

1. The P' waves are inverted and either appear before, after, or are hidden in QRS complexes.
2. The QRS duration is normal.
3. The P'–R interval will be less when P' waves appear before the QRS complex.

A junctional rhythm is called accelerated junctional rhythm when the rate is between 60 and 100 beats/min (Fig. 8.12). Rest of the features are same. In junctional tachycardia, the rate is more than 100 beats/min and rest of the features are like junctional rhythm (Fig. 8.13).

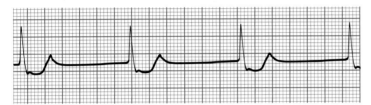

Fig 8.11   Junctional rhythm. Note that the P' waves are not seen as they are hidden in the QRS complexes. The QRS complexes are of normal duration. The rate is 48 beats/min.

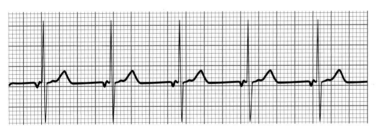

Fig 8.12   Accelerated junctional rhythm. Note the inverted P' waves before the QRS complexes and the heart rate is 79 beats/min.

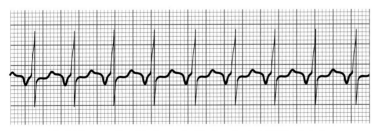

Fig 8.13   Junctional tachycardia. The heart rate is 136 beats/min.

VENTRICULAR ARRHYTHMIA

Ventricular arrhythmias originate from the ventricles. The electrical impulse does not follow normal pathway and depolarizes one ventricle before the other. The ventricular arrhythmias are thought to be due to altered automaticity, triggered activity, or re-entry. The common types of ventricular rhythm disturbances are the following:

1. Ventricular extrasystoles
2. Ventricular tachycardia (VT)
3. Ventricular flutter
4. Ventricular fibrillation (VF)
5. Idioventricular rhythm (IVR)
6. Accelerated idioventricular rhythm (AIVR)
7. Ventricular asystole

Ventricular Extrasystoles

Ventricular extrasystoles originate from the premature discharge of an ectopic focus either in the right or left ventricle. It is the commonest ventricular arrhythmia. It is usually seen in almost all types of heart disease. Sometimes it may be seen in normal persons but in them one should carefully investigate an underlying cardiac disease. The ventricular extrasystole may be unifocal (arising from single focus) or multifocal (arising form multiple foci). Digitalis is a frequent cause of ventricular extrasystoles. The various causes of ventricular extrasystoles are summarized in Box 8.4

Box 8.4   Causes of Ventricular Extrasystoles

- Coronary artery disease
- Digitalis toxicity
- Electrolyte imbalance
- Acid–base disturbance
- Congestive heart failure
- Hypoxia
- Acute myocardial infarction
- During or after reperfusion therapy or angioplasty
- Cardiac surgery
- Cardiomyopathy

The extrasystole arises from an irritable focus in the myocardium of the ventricle. This impulse then activates the ventricles and this impulse does not depolarize the SA node and hence, the sinus rhythm is maintained. However, the next sinus beat after the extrasystole will not be able to activate the ventricles because they are in a refractory state. The ventricle will respond to the next sinus impulse. This will lead to a pause, which is known as compensatory pause.

Ventricular extrasystole is diagnosed by the following features:

1. The beat arises prematurely, i.e., it occurs earlier than the anticipated QRS complex.
2. The P wave is absent in the extrasystoles.
3. The QRS complex is wide, bizarre with the S–T segment and T wave in opposite direction to the dominant QRS deflection. The duration of QRS complex is more than 0.12 s.
4. The compensatory pause is complete, i.e., the R–R interval between the two sinus beats preceding and following the ventricular extrasystoles is double the R–R interval between two normal sinus beats (Fig. 8.14a, b).

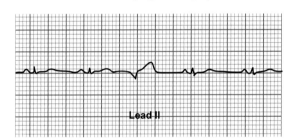

Fig 8.14a   Ventricular extrasystole. Note the wide and bizarre QRS complex.

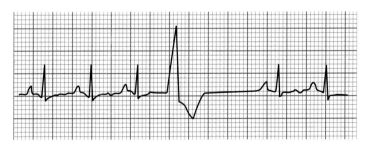

Fig 8.14b   Ventricular extrasystole. Note the wide and bizarre QRS complex. Also, note the complete compensatory pause.

When one ventricular extrasystole is present after every sinus beat, that is an alternation of sinus beat and ventricular extrasystole, this is called ventricular bigeminy (Fig. 8.14c). The classification used to assess the severity of ventricular extrasystoles is given in Box. 8.5.

Treatment
Ventricular extrasystoles are common findings in normal individuals and do not require active treatment in most of the cases. Precipitating factors and underlying causes should be treated. Beta-blockers and calcium channel blockers are required in some cases.

Ventricular Tachycardia
Ventricular tachycardia (VT) occurs due to rapid discharge from an ectopic ventricular focus. When three or more ventricular extrasystoles occur in rapid succession, it is known as VT. It is associated with severe myocardial disease and the commonest cause is ischaemic heart disease. It is also frequently seen in digitalis toxicity. VT is practically always an indicator of serious heart disease. It is very rarely seen in patients without any heart disease. It is a very serious arrhythmia and the underlying cause should be detected quickly

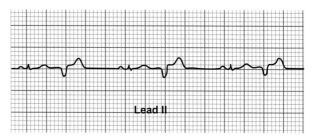

Lead II

Fig 8.14c   Ventricular bigeminy.

Box 8.5   Classification of Severity of Ventricular Extrasystoles
• Class 0: No ectopy
• Class 1: Less than 30 extrasystoles/hour
• Class 2: More than 30 extrasystoles/hour
• Class 3: Multiform complexes
• Class 4A: Couplets
• Class 4B: Runs of three or more
• Class 5: R on T phenomenon

and the arrhythmia should be treated on emergency basis. VT may lead to VF. The causes of VT are summarized in Box 8.6.

VT is often preceded by frequent ventricular extrasystoles. VT may be sustained (more than 30 s) or non-sustained (less than 30 s). The atrial rate is not discernable, ventricular rate is 100–250 beats/ min. P waves may be present or absent. If P waves are visible then it bears no relation with the QRS complex. The QRS complex is wide (greater than 0.12 s) and bizarre. The ventricular rate is usually regular. In VT, the QRS complexes in a single lead are similar in morphology and direction (concordance pattern) (Fig. 8.15a–c). Often it becomes difficult to differentiate between VT and SVT with intraventricular conduction defect. In this situation, the rhythm should be treated as VT until and unless proved otherwise.

The following characteristics suggest ventricular origin of the arrhythmia:

1. QRS duration > 0.14 s
2. AV dissociation with or without fusion and captured beat
3. Superior QRS axis in presence of right bundle branch block
4. Concordance of QRS pattern in all precordial leads, i.e., all positive or all negative waves

Box 8.6 Causes of Ventricular Tachycardia

- Acute myocardial infarction
- Digitalis toxicity
- Rheumatic heart disease
- Acid–base imbalance
- Electrolyte imbalance
- Catecholamines

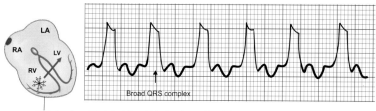

All the impulses originate in right ventricle at a rate more than 100 beats/minute

Fig 8.15a Illustration of genesis of ventricular tachycardia (VT). Note that the impulse is originating from a focus in right ventricle at a rate more than 100 beats/min. The impulses are not travelling via the normal conducting system resulting in broad complexes with bizarre shape.

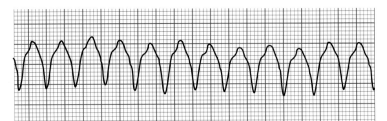

Fig 8.15b   VT. The ventricular premature complexes are occurring at a rate more than 100 beats/min.

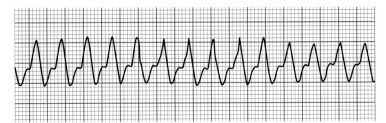

Fig 8.15c   VT. Note the wide QRS complexes occurring at a rate more than 100 beats/min.

The sinus beat and the ventricular beat is usually dissociated and they bear no relation with each other. The sinus impulse and the ventricular impulse meet with each other in the AV node and interfere with each other; thus, P waves bear no relation with QRS complex. This is called 'atrioventricular dissociation' (AV dissociation). Sometimes the atria may be retrogradely activated by ventricular impulse and then the QRS complex will be followed by a P' wave. This P' wave may be inverted in leads II, III, and aVF.

Capture Beat and Fusion Beat

Sometimes it may happen that a sinus impulse is able to travel into the ventricle via the AV node during its non-refractory phase. This impulse has the power to activate the ventricles in a normal fashion resulting in a normal QRS complex and this QRS complex is preceded by a normal P wave. This normal PQRS complex can be identified if the previous sinus rhythm is recorded in ECG. This beat in the presence of VT is called capture beat and is a reliable indicator of ventricular origin of the arrhythmia. Usually, only one capture beat is seen, between two ventricular extrasystoles during VT (Fig. 8.16).

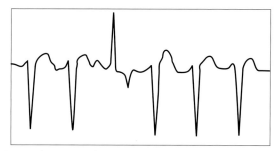

Fig 8.16 Capture beat. Note the normal QRS complex in between the ventricular extrasystoles. Capture beat is a confirmatory feature of ventricular origin of arrhythmia

Sometimes the capture beat may enter into the ventricles concomitantly with the ectopic ventricular impulse and in this case, the resulting beat will have the features of both capture beat and ventricular extrasystole, i.e., in between pure sinus beat and pure ventricular extrasystole. This beat is called 'fusion beat.' It is the most reliable indicator of ventricular origin of the arrhythmia.

Treatment

Lignocaine (1–1.5 mg/kg IV bolus) and procainamide are the most effective drugs in acute therapy especially when there is no haemodynamic compromise. Direct current (DC) cardioversion with high energy is required when pulse is absent. However, programmed stimulation is the best method to select appropriate therapy. Implanted cardioverter/defibrillator is often required in recurrent VT. VT with congenital long QT syndrome is treated with beta-blocker, calcium channel blocker, amiodarone etc.

Torsades de Pointes

This is a type of VT or ventricular flutter. The QRS complexes are of multiform type. It is also called polymorphic VT. Torsades de pointes means twisting or torsion of points. The QRS complexes have beat-to-beat variation or change in amplitude and direction. This gives an appearance of rotation of the QRS complexes around an isoelectric line (Fig. 8.17). It is usually associated with an underlying prolongation of Q–T interval, which favours VT.

Treatment

Beta-blocker and phenytoin (shortens Q–T interval) are the main stay of therapy. Metabolic abnormalities and drugs causing Torsades de pointes should be removed.

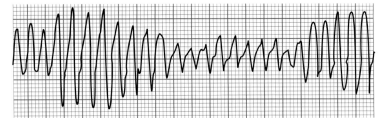

Fig 8.17   Torsades de pointes.

Ventricular Flutter and Fibrillation

Ventricular flutter occurs due to rapid and regular discharge from an ectopic ventricular focus. The QRS and T wave deflections are very broad, bizarre, and is often is difficult to separate the QRS complex, S–T segment, and the T wave. This is because of intraventricular conduction disturbance. The complexes are usually large in amplitude (Fig. 8.18).

Ventricular fibrillation occurs due to rapid and irregular discharge from an ectopic ventricular focus. This results in irregular, chaotic, deformed deflections of varying height and width (Fig. 8.19). In this condition, the ECG shows an undulating baseline with irregular waveforms that vary in morphology. VF with low amplitude waves

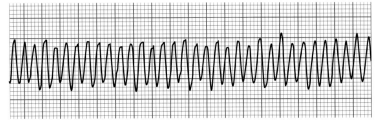

Fig 8.18   Ventricular flutter.

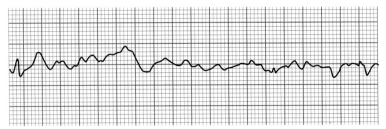

Fig 8.19   Ventricular fibrillation. Note that the complexes have no definite configuration. They are totally chaotic in nature.

Box 8.7 Causes of Ventricular Fibrillation

- Coronary artery disease
- Digitalis and quinidine toxicity
- Hypothermia
- Cardiac surgery
- Electric shock
- Electrolyte imbalance
- Acid–base disturbance
- Untreated ventricular tachycardia

(less than 3 mm) is called 'fine' VF whereas waves, which are more than 3 mm, are often called 'coarse' VF. The ventricular activation is chaotic and they are unable to respond properly to each stimulus. The coordinated muscle contraction is lost and thus, the patient looses the pulse and blood pressure.

VF is a very serious life threatening arrhythmia. It is seen in almost all the conditions associated with VT. The commonest cause is myocardial infarction and is the commonest cause of death within the first hour of infarction. Cardiac surgery, electric shock, and hypothermia may also cause VF. It should be immediately treated with DC shock. The various causes of VF are summarized in Box 8.7.

Treatment
Defibrillation ($\geq$200 Ws) is the main treatment of VF. Implanted cardioverter/defibrillator is indicated in those where recurrent VF is seen.

Idioventricular Rhythm
This is a type of ectopic rhythm that originates from an ectopic pacemaker located in the ventricular myocardium. The inherent ventricular rate is about 20–40 beats/min. It is considered to be an escape rhythm as it occurs when the rate of formation of impulse from SA node or the AV node becomes less than the pacemaker in the ventricles.

The QRS complexes are wide and bizarre, regular or may be slightly irregular and have no relation with atrial activity (Fig. 8.20).

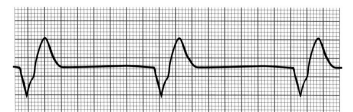

Fig 8.20   Idioventricular rhythm. Note the slow rate of extrasystoles at less than 40 beats/min.

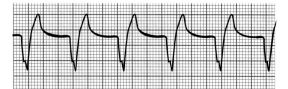

Fig 8.21   Accelerated idioventricular rhythm.

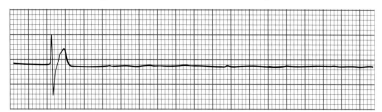

Fig 8.22:   Ventricular asystole. After one complex there is ventricular asystole.

Accelerated Idioventricular Rhythm

This also originates from an ectopic pacemaker located in the ventricle like IVR but the rate of generation of impulse is 50–100 beats/min. The term 'accelerated' means the rate is more than IVR but less than that of VT. It is also called slow VT. ECG is just like IVR, only the rate is more (Fig. 8.21).

AIVR is commonly seen after myocardial infarction and reperfusion therapy, digitalis toxicity, myocarditis, etc. AIVR can be treated by increasing the sinus rate with atropine but it is usually not required.

Ventricular Asystole

Ventricular asystole is also called ventricular standstill. There is no electrical activity in the ventricles. Most often in ECG it is manifested by a straight line (Fig. 8.22). It usually occurs after VF. The chance of revival is very low. Cardiopulmonary resuscitation must be started at the earliest.

APPROACH TO ARRHYTHMIA

There are various ways of approaching arrhythmia. The choice of course depends on the knowledge and the level of understanding of the reader. The easy method is to analyze by starting with the rate and regularity and then narrow down to the various possibilities. When analyzing by this method the following questions should be asked while inspecting the rhythm strip.

1. Is the rate normal, fast or slow?
2. Is the rhythm regular?
3. If the rhythm is irregular whether there is pattern of regularity to the rhythm that is regularly irregular or it is absolutely irregular that is irregularly irregular?
4. If there are only a few beats interrupting the regularity then it needs to be seen whether these are ectopic beats or whether these beats are followed by compensatory pause?

Now let us see the interpretation of these questions.

Consider the following possibilities when the rhythm is regular:

1. Normal rate
   a. Sinus rhythm (regular P waves present)
   b. Sinus rhythm absent (regular P waves absent)
      (i) Ectopic atrial pacemaker (P' wave present)
      (ii) Accelerated AV nodal rhythm
      (iii) Implanted pacemaker (ventricular)
2. Tachycardia
   a. Sinus tachycardia (P waves present, narrow QRS complex)
   b. PSVT/PAT (P waves usually not seen, narrow QRS complex)
   c. VT (P waves usually not seen, wide QRS complex)
3. Bradycardia
   a. Sinus bradycardia
   b. Idioventricular rhythm with SA block or complete AV block
   c. AV nodal rhythm with SA block or complete AV block

Consider the possibilities when the rhythm is irregular:

1. Regularly irregular arrhythmias
   a. Sinus arrhythmia

    b. Mobitz type I block (Wenckebach block)

    c. Bigeminy or trigeminy of atrial, AV nodal, or ventricular origin

2. Irregularly irregular arrhythmias

    a. Atrial flutter with variable AV block

    b. Atrial fibrillation

    c. VF

3. Infrequent irregularity

    a. Atrial, AV nodal or ventricular premature beats

    b. Mobitz type II AV block

Consider the following when there are pauses:

1. Long pause

    a. Sinus pause

    b. Complete AV block with failure of escape beat

2. Short pause

    a. Ventricular ectopic (complete pause)

    b. Atrial ectopic (incomplete pause)

Another method of analysing arrhythmias is by the study of the P wave and its relation with the QRS complexes. Here, initially it has to be seen whether sinus rhythm is present or not. If the sinus rhythm is absent, then the number and the morphology of the P waves are to be studied and then the irregularities of the P waves are to be correlated with the QRS complexes. It is always better to mark out all the P waves in the rhythm strip at the beginning. The duration of the QRS complex should also be measured because a wide QRS complex points towards the ventricular origin of the arrhythmia. Let us consider the following:

1. Sinus rhythm

    a. Regular sinus rhythm

    b. Sinus bradycardia

    c. Sinus tachycardia

    d. Sinus arrhythmia

2. Absent sinus rhythm

    a. Absent P waves

      (i) Infrequent absence

        • Ventricular ectopic

        • Premature beat of nodal origin

      (ii) Constant absence of P wave (or P wave buried in T wave)

- Atrial fibrillation
- VT
- Nodal rhythm
- Accelerated nodal rhythm
- PSVT

b. Abnormal shape of P wave (P' wave)
  (i) Atrial ectopic beat
  (ii) Wandering atrial pacemaker
  (iii) Incorrect placement of arm electrodes
  (iv) Nodal rhythm with retrograde conduction of P waves

c. More than one P wave for each QRS complex
  (i) Complete AV block
  (ii) 2:1 or higher AV block (Mobitz type I and II)
  (iii) Atrial flutter or fibrillation with second degree AV block (very difficult to identify P wave in these cases)

One can use either of these methods alone or together to analyse arrhythmia but it is easier said than done because analysis of arrhythmia is one of the most difficult aspect of ECG. This comes not by reading book alone, but by constant daily practice.

BIBLIOGRAPHY

1. Akhtar M. Supraventricular tachycardias. Electrophysiologic mechanisms: Diagnosis and pharmacological therapy, in Josephson ME and Wellens HJ (eds), *Tachycardias: Mechanisms, Diagnosis, Treatment*. Lea & Febiger: Philadelphia, PA, 1984: p. 137.

2. Alpert MA, Mukerji V, Bikkina M, et al. Pathogenesis, recognition, and management of common cardiac arrhythmias. Part I: ventricular premature beats and tachyarrhythmias. *South Med J* 1995; 88(1), 1–21.

3. Belhassen B and Viskin S. Idiopathic ventricular tachycardia and fibrillation. *J Cardiovasc Electrophysiol* 1993; 4(3), 356–368.

4. Bonnemeier H, Ortak J, Wiegand UK, et al. Accelerated idioventricular rhythm in the post-thrombolytic era: incidence, prognostic implications, and modulating mechanisms after direct percutaneous coronary intervention. *Ann Noninvasive Electrocardiol* 2005; 10(2), 179–187.

5. Braunwald E. Heart Disease: A Textbook of Cardiovascular Medicine, Fifth edition, W.B. Saunders Co.: Philadelphia, PA, 1997; pp. 641–656.

6. Chen PS, Athill CA, Wu TJ, et al. Mechanisms of atrial fibrillation and flutter and implications for management. *Am J Cardiol* 1999; 84(9A), 125R–130R.

7. Childers R. Teaching electrocardiogram interpretation. *J Electrocardiol* 2006; 39(4), 426–429.

8. Davidenko JM and Snyder LS. Causes of errors in the electrocardiographic diagnosis of atrial fibrillation by physicians. *J Electrocardiol* 2007; 40(5), 450–456.

9. Demas E, Sallyann J and Francis M. ABC of clinical electrocardiography: junctional tachycardias. *BMJ* 2002; 324, 662–665.

10. Farre J and Wellens HJ. The value of the electrocardiogram in diagnosing site of origin and mechanism of supraventricular tachycardia, in Wellens HJJ and Kulbetus HE (eds), *What's New in Electrocardiography*. Martinus Nijhoff: The Hague, Belgium, 1981; pp. 131–171.

11. Goodacre S and Irons R. ABC of clinical electrocardiography: atrial arrhythmias. *BMJ* 2002; 324(7337), 594–597.

12. Hohnloser SH, Kuck KH and Lilienthal J. Rhythm or rate control in atrial fibrillation—pharmacological intervention in atrial fibrillation (PIAF): a randomised trial. *Lancet* 2000; 356(9244), 1789–1794.

13. Jais P, Shah DC, Haissaguerre M, et al. Atrial fibrillation: role of arrhythmogenic foci. *J Interv Card Electrophysiol* 2000; 4(Suppl 1), 29–37.

14. June E and Francis M. ABC of clinical electrocardiography: broad complex tachycardia—Part I. *BMJ* 2002; 324, 719–722.

15. June E and Francis M. ABC of clinical electrocardiography: broad complex tachycardia—Part II. *BMJ* 2002; 324, 776–779.

16. Prystowsky EN, Benson DW Jr, Fuster V et al. Management of patients with atrial fibrillation. A statement for healthcare professionals. From the Subcommittee on Electrocardiography and Electrophysiology, American Heart Association. *Circulation* 1996; 93(6), 1262–1277.

17. Steve G and Richard I. ABC of clinical electrocardiography: atrial arrhythmias. *BMJ* 2002; 324, 594–597.

18. Wilde AAM. Arrhythmias and the electrocardiogram in inherited arrhythmia disorders. *J Electrocardiol* 2007; 40(1), S7–S8.

19 Xie B, Thakur RK, Shah CP, et al. Clinical differentiation of narrow QRS complex tachycardias. *Emerg Med Clin North Am* 1998; 16(2), 295–330.

CHAPTER 9

Effect of Drugs and Electrolytes on ECG

Chapter Outline

INTRODUCTION

Drugs and electrolyte imbalance cause several changes in the electro-cardiogram (ECG). In this chapter some of the common abnormalities that we frequently observe will be discussed.

EFFECT OF DRUGS ON ECG

Effects of Digitalis

Digitalis is one of the commonest drugs to produce changes in ECG. Digitalis is water soluble and is highly concentrated in the myocardium. It influences the repolarization of myocardium. The serum level of digitalis, at a standard dose, in which no toxicity is seen is 1.0–1.5 ng/ml. The ECG change produced at this level is called digitalis effect. The ECG changes are:

1. S–T segment depression
2. Decrease in magnitude of T wave
3. Decrease in Q–T interval

S–T Segment Depression

The S–T segment is depressed. The 'j' point (junction between R or S wave and S–T segment) remains at isoelectric level. After that the S–T segment slopes downwards with a sharp terminal rise and blends with the T wave. This produces the mirror image of a correction mark (Figs. 9.1a, b and 9.2). The S–T segment often has a scooped configuration. If the 'j' point is also depressed it indicates digitalis toxicity.

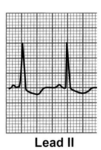

Lead II

Fig. 9.1a   Digitalis effect.

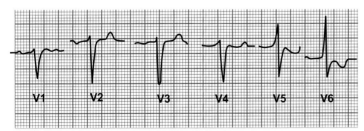

Fig. 9.1b   Digitalis effect. Note the reverse check sign in leads V5 and V6.

Decrease in Magnitude of T Wave

In digitalis effect, the T wave is slightly diminished in magnitude but the direction remains unchanged. Along with a depressed S–T segment often the T wave appears to be dragged down. In digitalis toxicity, the amplitude of T wave is decreased and often it is inverted. However, it should be kept in mind that the T wave may be inverted due to pre-existing coronary artery disease. In digitalis effect, the T wave is depressed and rises above the baseline before becoming isoelectric, but in digitalis toxicity the T wave does not rise above the baseline (Fig. 9.2). Sometimes digitalis may cause slight increase in the amplitude of U wave.

Decrease in Q–T Interval

Digitalis decreases the duration of electrical systole. The Q–T interval is shortened in digitalis effect because the refractory period of ventricular myocardium is shortened.

Digitalis Toxicity

Digitalis toxicity is a very common toxicity that we often see in our routine practice. The serum level of digitalis is usually more than 2–3 ng/ml when the features of toxicity appear in the ECG. Hypokalaemia due to diuretic therapy is one of the most common factors that precipitates digitalis toxicity. The various ECG changes are as follows:

S–T Segment Depression

There is down sloping S–T segment depression like digitalis effect, but along with it there is depression of the j point also, and there is no terminal positivity of the inverted T wave (Fig. 9.2). The T wave does not rise above the baseline.

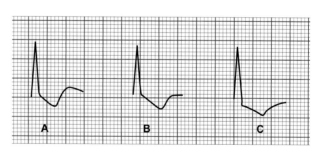

Fig. 9.2   Diagrams of digitalis toxicity and digitalis effect. (A) Reverse check sign. Note the terminal positivity of the T wave. (B) Digitalis toxicity. Note that the terminal part of the T wave does not rise above the baseline. (C) Digitalis toxicity. Note that the terminal part of the T wave does not rise above the baseline. It can also be due to primary T wave abnormality because of coronary artery disease.

Cardiac Arrhythmia

Almost any type of cardiac arrhythmia is seen in digitalis toxicity. However, type II second-degree atrioventricular (AV) block is not seen. The arrhythmias commonly seen are sinus bradycardia, first-degree AV block, ventricular extrasystoles (uniform and multiform), and ventricular bigeminy. Wenckebach type of block may be seen. Complete heart block, sino-atrial (SA) block, AV dissociation, AV junctional rhythm, and ventricular fibrillation may be observed sometimes. Nonparoxysmal atrial tachycardia with variable AV block is characteristic of digitalis toxicity. The various ECG changes in digitalis toxicity are summarized in Box 9.1.

Digitalis toxicity is manifested by anorexia, nausea, vomiting, yellow vision etc. The toxicity commonly occurs because of a narrow therapeutic window. Toxicity is seen when serum level exceeds 2 ng/ml. Co-administration of quinidine, verapamil, amiodarone, and propafenone predisposes to toxicity.

Digitalis toxicity is treated by stopping digitalis and by treating hypokalaemia. Potassium should be given orally. Intravenous lignocaine, phenytoin sodium, temporary pacing may be required. Purified Fab fragments are given in severe life threatening toxicity.

Quinidine Effect

Quinidine is a class Ia antiarrhythmic drug. It is a cardiac depressant. It is mainly used in the management of atrial arrhythmias. It decreases the rate of ectopic discharge and then eliminates the ectopic generation and allows resumption of normal rhythm. It has vagolytic effect, which increases the rate of conduction through the AV node. Thus, it can potentially increase the ventricular rate and

Box 9.1   Changes in Digitalis Toxicity
• S–T segment depression (including 'j' point depression)
• T wave inversion
• Sinus bradycardia
• Uniform or multiform ventricular extrasystoles
• Ventricular tachycardia, flutter, and fibrillation
• Paroxysmal atrial tachycardia
• Atrial flutter and fibrillation
• Sino-atrial block
• Bundle branch block
• First, second, and third degree AV block

hence, it is always better to digitalize the patient before starting quinidine. Quinidine produces the following ECG changes:

1. Prolongation of Q–T interval: The prolongation of Q–T interval is due to prolongation of repolarization. This is in contrast to digitalis toxicity (Fig. 9.3).

2. *Prolongation of QRS complex:* QRS complex may be widened up to 50% or even more, and an increase over 40% is an indication to stop quinidine therapy. This widening contributes to prolongation of Q–T interval. The widening occurs because quinidine causes depression of intraventricular conduction. The QRS complex maintains its shape. Quinidine may also cause right or left bundle branch block and lead to widening of QRS complex.

3. *Prominent U wave:* There may be slight prominence of U wave.

4. *Mild prolongation of P–R interval:* The P–R interval may be prolonged. It is usually not marked and it is not an indication for stopping quinidine therapy.

5. *S–T segment depression:* The depression of S–T segment is usually rare and mild. There is no particular configuration of S–T segment depression. This· is best seen in lead V5 or V6.

6. *T wave widening and inversion.*

7. *P wave may be wide and notched.*

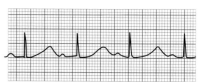

Remember toxicity of digitalis together with quinidine resembles hypokalaemia. The toxic effects of quinidine on ECG are summarized in Box 9.2.

Fig. 9.3   Quinidine toxicity. Note the prolongation of the Q–T interval. Note also the prolongation of the P–R interval. Usually it is mild but sometimes it may be significantly prolonged.

Box 9.2   Toxic Effects of Quinidine on ECG

- First, second, and third degree AV block
- Left and right bundle branch block
- Sino-atrial block
- Ventricular arrhythmias
- AV dissociation

Effects of Emetine

Emetine produces the following ECG changes:

1. Widening of P–R interval
2. S–T segment depression
3. T wave inversion
4. Intraventricular conduction disturbances

Effects of Tricyclic Antidepressant

Tricyclic antidepressants are myocardial depressants and may cause conduction disturbances. The ECG changes are:

1. S–T segment depression
2. T wave inversion
3. Q–T interval prolongation
4. Prominent U wave
5. Atrioventricular and intraventricular conduction disturbances

Effects of Anthracycline Antibiotics

The anthracycline antibiotics are doxorubicin and daunorubicin. These are chemotherapeutic agents. These are cardiotoxic and cause diffuse T wave inversion.

EFFECT OF ELECTROLYTE IMBALANCE ON ECG

Electrolyte abnormality is frequently seen in our day-to-day practice. It is commonly seen in patients who are severely ill, patients on IV fluids, patients suffering from renal failure, as side effect of drugs such as frusemide. In this section, only the commonly encountered ECG abnormalities due to electrolyte imbalances will be discussed.

Hyperkalaemia

Hyperkalaemia means serum potassium level is more than the upper limit of normal (more than 5.5 mEq/l). However, the ECG changes are mainly seen when the serum potassium level is more than 6 mEq/l. The various ECG changes of hyperkalaemia are:

1. *Peaked, tall, and tented T waves:* Peaked, tall, and tented T wave is the earliest feature of hyperkalaemia. This is seen best in the precordial leads. At first, the T wave becomes tall and then becomes slightly wide. This is called 'tented' T wave. This is seen when serum potassium is usually more than 6.8 mEq/l (Fig. 9.4a–d).

2. *Gradual decrease and then disappearance of P wave:* The prolongation of P–R interval may precede the disappearance of
P wave. The P wave disappears because the atria are not activated though the SA node fires and the impulse travels via the
internodal pathways to the AV node. The P wave usually disappears when serum potassium level is more than 7.5 mEq/l.

3. *Widening of QRS complexes:* The QRS complex becomes
wide and bizarre in shape. This mainly affects the terminal
deflection. This conduction disturbance resembles bundle
branch block. This picture is seen when serum potassium is
usually more than 9.1 mEq/l.

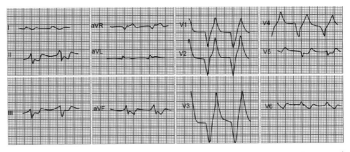

Fig. 9.4a ECG showing hyperkalaemia. Note the wide QRS complexes and
tall T waves. At this time, the serum potassium level was 9.1mEq/l. Calcium glu-
conate injection was administered and insulin glucose drip was started.

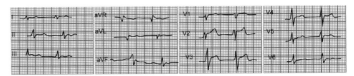

Fig. 9.4b ECG of the same patient after correction of serum potassium.

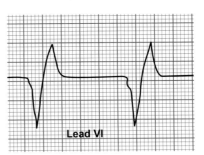

Fig. 9.4c Hyperkalaemia showing sine wave configuration of the QRS complex.

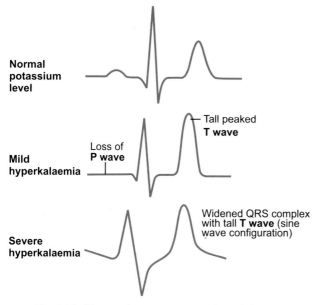

Normal potassium level

Mild hyperkalaemia

Loss of **P wave**

Tall peaked **T wave**

Severe hyperkalaemia

Widened QRS complex with tall **T wave** (sine wave configuration)

Fig. 9.4d   Diagram showing progressive hyperkalaemia.

4. *Virtual disappearance of S–T segment:* With rise in serum potassium level, the S–T segment virtually disappears as if the proximal limb is incorporated in the ascending limb of T wave.
5. AV conduction defect.
6. Ventricular tachycardia and fibrillation.
7. Q–T interval is normal or decreased.

Hyperkalaemia is treated by withdrawing potassium containing food and drinks, intravenous infusion of insulin and glucose, intravenous bicarbonate, etc. Potassium exchange resins and haemodialysis are used in severe hyperkalaemia.

Hypokalaemia

Hypokalaemia means serum potassium level is less than 3 mEq/l. Hypokalaemia is commonly seen in patients receiving diuretics, prolonged IV fluid therapy, vomiting, diarrhoea, etc. The gradual fall in serum potassium level is reflected electrocardiographically by the following features:

1. *Gradual decrease and then disappearance of T wave:* The T wave gradually becomes flat and then disappears. Later it may be seen as a small hump on the S–T segment.

2. *Presence of prominent U waves, best seen in leads V2–V4:* With the fall in serum potassium level the U wave becomes prominent. When the T wave has disappeared the U wave may give a false impression of T wave. Thus, it may also lead to an appearance of Q–T interval prolongation, which is basically a Q–U interval. The U wave maintains its round shape (Figs. 9.5 and 9.6).

3. *Slight depression of S–T segment:* There may be S–T segment depression in all the leads.

4. *Increase in P–R interval:* The P–R interval gradually increases and the P wave falls almost on the preceding U wave. Wenckebach type of second-degree block is usually seen with very low level of serum potassium.

Hypokalaemia is treated by oral or intravenous replacement of potassium. The cause of hypokalaemia should be treated. Intravenous potassium should always be very carefully monitored.

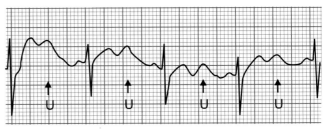

Fig. 9.5   Hypokalaemia.

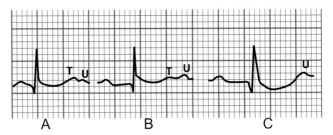

Fig. 9.6   Diagram showing progressive changes in hypokalaemia. (A) Normal complex. (B) Hypokalaemia. Note the prominence of U wave, which is taller than the T wave. The P–R interval is prolonged. (C) With further fall in serum potassium level, the U wave becomes very prominent with disappearance of the T wave. Note the further prolongation of the P–R interval.

Hypocalcaemia

The normal serum calcium level is 9–10.5 mg/dl. Hypocalcaemia occurs when the serum level of calcium is below the lower limit of normal. It is manifested by prolongation of Q–T interval. The increase in Q–T interval is due to increase in the S–T segment, which is due to prolongation of phase 2 of action potential. However, the S–T segment is not displaced. The Q–T interval may be in the region of 0.5–0.6 s (Fig. 9.7). The T wave may rarely become inverted or tall.

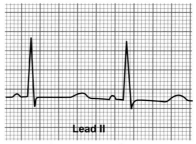

Fig. 9.7 Hypocalcaemia.

Hypercalcaemia

The ECG changes usually appear when the serum calcium level is more than 12 mg/dl. It is manifested by shortening of Q–T interval which is due to the shortening of S–T segment. This occurs due to the shortening of the phase 2 of action potential. The S–T segment virtually disappears and gets incorporated in the T wave as if it forms the proximal limb of T wave (Fig. 9.8). At serum level of calcium above 16 mg% or more, the T wave may be prolonged and may also be flattened.

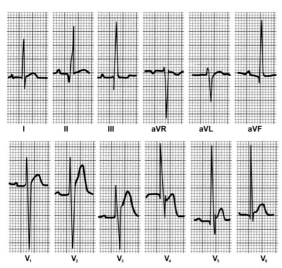

Fig. 9.8 Hypercalcaemia. Note the shortened Q–T interval.

Effect of Magnesium

Usually, the serum potassium and magnesium go hand in hand and the ECG changes are also similar. The ECG changes of hypomagnesaemia resembles that of hypokalaemia. The U wave increases and the T wave becomes flattened. The S–T segment may be depressed.

The ECG changes of hypermagnesaemia resemble that of hyperkalaemia. There may be widening of QRS complex and increase of the P–R interval.

BIBLIOGRAPHY

1. Bassett AL and Hoffman BF. Antiarrhythmic drugs: electrophysiological actions. *Annu Rev Pharmacol* 1971; 11, 143–170.
2. Douglas PS, Carmichael KA and Palevsky PM. Extreme hypercalcemia and electrocardiographic changes. *Am J Cardiol* 1984; 54(6), 674–675.
3. Elkayam U and Frishman W. Cardiovascular effects of phenothiazines. *Am Heart J* 1980; 100, 397–401.
4. Fisch C. Relation of electrolyte disturbances to cardiac arrhythmias. *Circulation* 1973; 47, 408–419.
5. Fisch C and Knoebl SB. Recognition and therapy of digitalis toxicity. *Prog Cardiovasc Dis* 1970; 13, 71–96.
6. Garberoglio L, Giustetto C, Wolpert C, et al. Is acquired short QT due to digitalis intoxication responsible for malignant ventricular arrhythmias? *J Electrocardiol* 2007; 40(1), 43–46.
7. Langer GA. Effects of digitalis on myocardial ionic exchange. *Circulation* 1972; 46(1), 180–187.
8. Schamroth L. *An Introduction to Electrocardiography*, Seventh edition, Blackwell Science (Indian Reprint), 2002; pp. 241–253.
9. Littmann L, Taylor L and Brearley WD Jr. ST-segment elevation: A common finding in severe hypercalcemia. *J Electrocardiol* 2007; 40(1), 60–62.
10. Surawicz B. Electrolytes and the electrocardiogram. *Am J Cardiol* 1963; 12, 656–662.

Miscellaneous Abnormal ECG

INTRODUCTION

In this chapter, electrocardiogram (ECG) changes of some common diseases will be discussed. It is very important to understand the changes, as ECG is often the first investigation for these diseases that help us in making the diagnosis before the treatment can be started.

ACUTE PULMONARY EMBOLISM

Acute pulmonary embolism is characterized by sudden onset of chest pain and dyspnoea. There is sudden right ventricular strain. Often these patients suffer from various types of cardiac arrhythmias. It is diagnosed electrocardiographically by the following criteria:

1. SI, QIII, TIII pattern, i.e., prominent S wave in lead I, Q wave in lead III, and T wave inversion in lead III (Fig. 10.1)
2. Right axis deviation
3. S–T segment depression in leads I and II
4. Tall-peaked P waves may appear in lead II
5. T inversion in leads V1–V3 due to right ventricular ischaemia
6. Low-voltage complexes
7. Right bundle branch block (RBBB)
8. Atrial arrhythmias

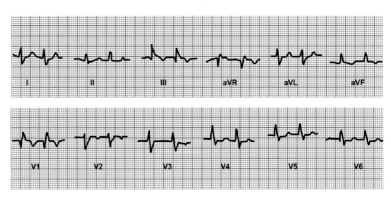

Fig. 10.1 Pulmonary embolism. There is sinus tachycardia with T wave inversion in leads V1 and V2. Note the SI, QIII, and TIII pattern.

CHRONIC OBSTRUCTIVE PULMONARY DISEASE

Chronic obstructive pulmonary disease (COPD) is a very common disease. Patients often present with acute exacerbation. In long standing cases, there is right ventricular hypertrophy (RVH) with pulmonary hypertension. There is right atrial enlargement as well. These patients often suffer from rhythm disturbances and conduction disturbances.

The ECG manifestations are:

1. P-pulmonale (height of P wave greater than 2.5 mm), best seen in leads II, III, and aVF (Fig. 10.2)

2. Clockwise rotation

3. Right axis deviation

4. RVH (R:S ratio greater than 1 in lead V1)

5. Decreased amplitude of QRS complexes

6. Incomplete or complete RBBB (rSR' complex in lead V1 with S–T segment, T wave change, and QRS duration greater than 0.12 s)

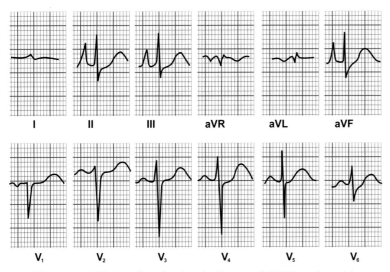

Fig. 10.2   COPD. Note the tall and peaked P wave of COPD (p-pulmonale).

MITRAL STENOSIS

Mitral stenosis is usually of rheumatic origin. There is left atrial hypertrophy and RVH. In long standing cases there is right atrial enlargement. Pulmonary hypertension is commonly observed in these patients. They often suffer from atrial fibrillation (Fig. 10.3). The various ECG manifestations of mitral stenosis are:

1. P-mitrale in lead II and biphasic P wave in lead V1

2. P-pulmonale is present in mitral stenosis with pulmonary artery hypertension

3. Features of RVH (R:S ratio greater than 1 in lead V1 with S–T segment, T wave change)

4. Right axis deviation

5. Presence of atrial fibrillation (absence of P wave with varying R–R interval)

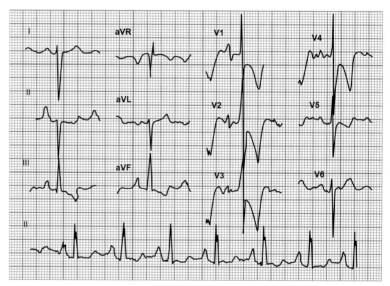

Fig. 10.3   Mitral stenosis. This ECG is recorded from a 17-year-old boy suffering from pure mitral stenosis. Note the tall R waves in lead V1 with small S waves and S–T segment, T wave changes suggestive of gross right ventricular hypertrophy. Note the biphasic P wave in leads V1 and V2, and tall P wave in lead II. Also note the widening of P wave in lead I.

MITRAL REGURGITATION

Mitral regurgitation is due to several causes such as rheumatic heart disease, dilated cardiomyopathy, mitral valve prolapse. There is left ventricular and left atrial hypertrophy. Pulmonary hypertension is usually absent. Atrial fibrillation may be seen. The ECG manifestations are:

1. Left atrial enlargement (deep and prominent negative component of biphasic P wave in lead V1)
2. Left ventricular hypertrophy due to diastolic overload (S in lead V1 plus R in lead V5 or V6 is greater than 35 mm, with S–T segment, T wave change in lead V5 or V6)
3. Normal QRS axis
4. Atrial fibrillation (absence of P wave with varying R–R interval)

AORTIC STENOSIS

In aortic stenosis, there is concentric hypertrophy of left ventricle. There is systolic overload of the left ventricle. The ECG features are:

1. Left ventricular hypertrophy (S in lead V1 plus R in lead V5 or V6 is greater than 35 mm, with S–T segment, T wave change in lead V5 or V6)
2. Normal QRS axis
3. Incomplete left bundle branch block (rSr' complex in lead V5 or V6 with QRS duration less than 0.12 s)
4. Left atrial enlargement
5. Inversion of U wave

AORTIC REGURGITATION

Aortic regurgitation is often of rheumatic origin. There is volume overload of the left ventricle. There is gross hypertrophy of the left ventricle. The left atrium is also enlarged. The ECG manifestations are:

1. Left ventricular hypertrophy (diastolic overload pattern)
2. Left atrial enlargement
3. Usually normal QRS axis, sometimes left anterior hemiblock may be seen
4. Sometimes inversion of U wave is seen

ACUTE RHEUMATIC CARDITIS

Acute rheumatic carditis occurs during acute rheumatic fever. Myocardium, pericardium, and endocardium are involved. The ECG manifestations of acute rheumatic carditis are:

1. Prolonged P–R interval
2. Sinus tachycardia
3. Features of acute pericarditis
4. Features of acute myocarditis
   - Depression or elevation of the S–T segment
   - Notching or slurring of the QRS complex
   - Non-specific T wave changes
   - Prolonged Q–T$_c$ interval

PERICARDITIS

Pericarditis may be of viral or bacterial origin. Tuberculous pericarditis is also very common. It is often associated with pericardial effusion. Uraemia is also an important cause of pericarditis. Acute pericarditis is diagnosed by the following ECG features:

1. Sinus tachycardia
2. S–T segment elevation with upward concavity in leads oriented towards the affected surface (Fig. 10.4)
3. T wave inversion (this occurs after the S–T segment becomes isoelectric)
4. Sometimes depression of the P–R segment is seen

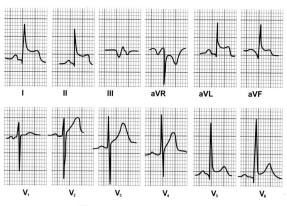

Fig. 10.4   Acute pericarditis.

PERICARDIAL EFFUSION

There are several causes of pericardial effusion. Tuberculosis, uraemia, viral pericarditis, etc. are some of the common causes. There is accumulation of fluid in the pericardial sac that compresses the heart often leading to cardiac tamponade. The ECG features of pericardial effusion are:

1. Low-voltage complex (less than 5 mm amplitude in standard leads and less than 10 mm amplitude in chest leads; see Fig. 10.5)
2. T wave inversion in most of the leads except aVR
3. Electrical alternans (alternating low and normal voltage QRS complexes)

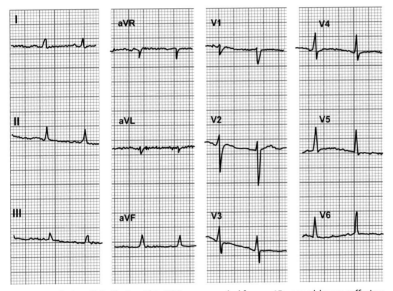

Fig. 10.5 Pericardial effusion. This ECG was recorded from a 45-year-old man suffering from tubercular effusion. Note the low-voltage complexes with sinus tachycardia.

ATRIAL SEPTAL DEFECT

Atrial septal defect (ASD) is of two types, viz., ostium secundum and ostium primum. Ostium secundum defect is not associated with any malformation of the atrioventricular (AV) canal. In this defect, there is volume overload of right atrium and right ventricle

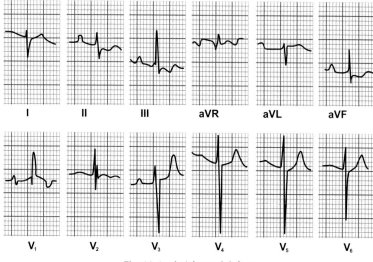

Fig. 10.6   Atrial septal defect.

(Fig. 10.6). The ECG features of ostium secundum type of ASD are the following:

1. rsR' complex in lead V1 with biphasic P wave
2. Right axis deviation
3. Right atrial enlargement
4. Decrease in amplitude of R wave in leads V5 and V6
5. Atrial fibrillation and atrial flutter may be observed
6. Clockwise electric rotation: the transition zone is shifted to lead V5 or V6

Ostium primum defect is often associated with malformation of AV canal. The ECG features of ostium primum type of ASD are:

1. rsR' complex in lead V1
2. Left axis deviation
3. First-degree AV block
4. Atrial arrhythmias

VENTRICULAR SEPTAL DEFECT

The ventricular septum is made up of a membranous part and a muscular part. Most of the defects lie in the membranous part of the interventricular septum. The muscular part is rarely affected.

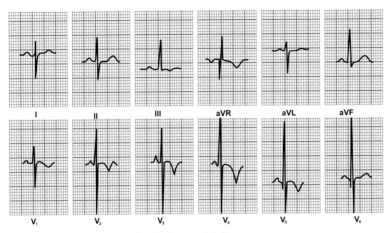

Fig. 10.7   Ventricular septal defect.

There is left to right shunt. There is volume overloading of the left atrium and the left ventricle. Due to gradual increase in the pulmonary resistance there is an increase in the right ventricular pressure, i.e., systolic overload. In the later stages there may be reversal of shunt resulting in Eisenmenger complex. The ECG features of ventricular septal defect (VSD) are the following:

1. Prominent q waves in leads II, III, and aVF
2. Features of left ventricular hypertrophy or combined left and right ventricular hypertrophy
3. Large amplitude equiphasic QRS deflections in leads V2–V4 (Fig. 10.7)
4. QRS axis is normal but with the development of pulmonary hypertension there may be right axis deviation

FALLOT'S TETRALOGY

Fallot's tetralogy is the commonest congenital cyanotic heart disease among adults. The four defects in the heart are (a) infundibular pulmonary stenosis, (b) dextroposition of aorta, (c) VSD, and (d) RVH. The ECG features of Fallot's tetralogy are:

1. RVH due to systolic overload (Fig. 10.8)
2. Tall and peaked P waves in lead II due to right atrial enlargement

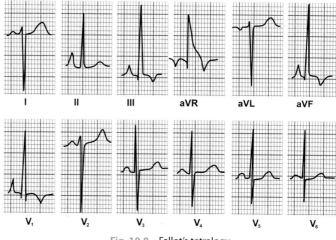

Fig. 10.8   Fallot's tetralogy.

PENTALOGY OF FALLOT

In this rare condition, there are all the features of tetralogy along with ostium secundum ASD. There is volume overloading of left atrium and left ventricle. Thus, there is enlargement of all the cardiac chambers. The ECG features consist of right atrial enlargement with RVH (systolic overload) and mild left ventricular hypertrophy (diastolic overload).

TRILOGY OF FALLOT

Trilogy of Fallot is pulmonary stenosis (valvular) with any of the following types of interatrial septal defect: (a) patent foramen ovale, (b) ostium secundum ASD, and (c) ostium primum ASD. The ECG features are:

1. RVH
2. RVH due to systolic overload
3. Possible left atrial and left ventricular hypertrophy

MYXOEDEMA

In myxoedema, body metabolism is decreased. There may be pericardial effusion. The ECG features of myxoedema are:

1. Low-voltage complex (Fig. 10.9)
2. Sinus bradycardia

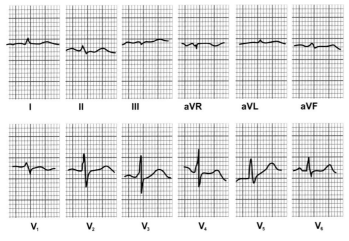

Fig. 10.9   Myxoedema.

3. Shallow or inverted T waves
4. Prolonged P–R interval

HYPOTHERMIA

Hypothermia is mainly due to exposure to cold air or water for a long time. Osborne wave or 'J' wave is the characteristic finding of hypothermia. Ventricular fibrillation may be seen when the core temperature falls below 28°C. The ECG features of hypothermia are:

1. Presence of 'J' waves (Fig. 10.10)
2. Prolongation of P–R, QRS, and Q–T intervals
3. Atrial fibrillation
4. Sinus bradycardia
5. AV junctional rhythm
6. Ventricular fibrillation may occur

MYOCARDITIS

Myocarditis is acute inflammation of the myocardium. Almost any acute infectious disease may involve the myocardium. Myocarditis may be due to viral or bacterial origin. It is very frequently a part of rheumatic fever. The ECG features are:

1. S–T segment, T wave changes in chest leads
2. First-degree heart block or defective intraventricular conduction

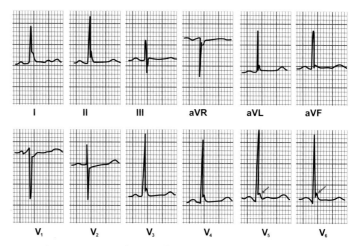

Fig. 10.10   Hypothermia. The J waves are shown with an arrow.

3. Prolongation of Q–Tc interval
4. Various types of arrhythmias
5. QRS abnormalities that may mimic myocardial infarction

HYPERTHYROIDISM

Hyperthyroidism is due to the presence and effect of excess circulating thyroid hormones. The body metabolism is increased and therefore there is tachycardia, which is a cardinal feature of hyperthyroidism. The ECG features are:

1. Sinus tachycardia
2. S–T segment, T wave change in left ventricular chest leads
3. Atrial and ventricular extrasystoles
4. Atrial fibrillation

DEXTROCARDIA

Dextrocardia is congenital malposition of heart. The left ventricle and left atrium is present in the right side of right ventricle and right atrium. The right atrium is on the left side and the aortic knob is on the right side. The ECG features of dextrocardia are:

1. Inverted P waves in leads I and aVL
2. QRS complexes are upright in leads II, III, and aVF
3. QRS complexes are negative in leads I and aVL

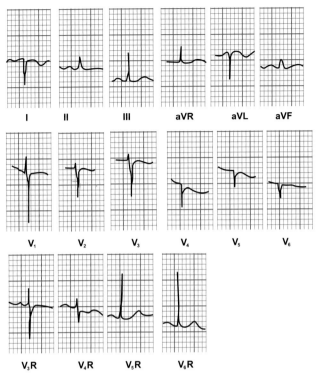

Fig. 10.11 Dextrocardia. Note the negative complexes in lead aVL and the positive complexes in lead aVR.

4. The P, QRS, and T waves in aVL resemble that of aVR and vice versa (Fig. 10.11)
5. R wave is prominent in lead V1 and the height of R wave gradually diminishes in lead V6, because the lead V1 overlies left ventricle and the lead V6 overlies right ventricle
6. The P, QRS, and T waves in leads V4R and V5R resemble that of leads V4 and V5
7. The QRS axis is the mirror image of the normal QRS axis (+60°) i.e., +120°

DEXTROVERSION

Dextroversion is congenital malposition of heart. The heart is displaced to right and the ventricles are rotated in counter clockwise direction. The ventricles and the atria are not transposed. The aorta is in normal position. QRS vector is directed more anteriorly

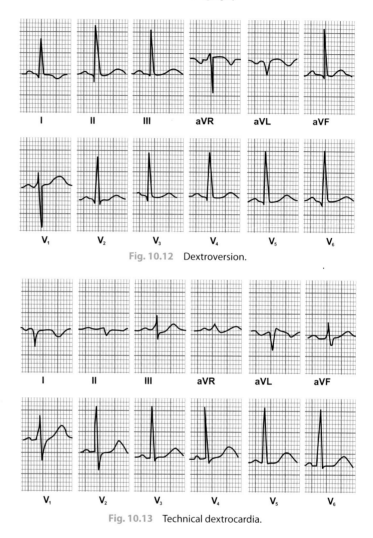

Fig. 10.12   Dextroversion.

Fig. 10.13   Technical dextrocardia.

because of counter clockwise rotation of the heart. The T wave is inverted in lead I (Fig. 10.12).

TECHNICAL DEXTROCARDIA

Technical dextrocardia is the term used when ECG is recorded by mistake in which the right and the left arm electrodes are interchanged with each other. There are features of dextrocardia in limb leads. The recordings in chest leads are normal (see Fig. 10.13).

PRE-EXCITATION SYNDROME (WOLF-PARKINSON-WHITE SYNDROME)

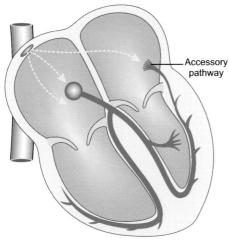

Accessory pathway

Fig. 10.14a   The accessory pathway.

Wolf–Parkinson–White syndrome (WPW) is the prototype of pre-excitation syndrome. This electrocardiographic syndrome is mainly due to an anomalous atrio-ventricular pathway or the accessory pathway (Fig. 10.14a). This pathway is of congenital origin and bypasses the AV node. This accessory pathway is known as Bundle of Kent. The syndrome is commonly associated with Ebstein's anomaly and hypertrophic cardiomyopathy.

The ECG of WPW syndrome has the following features:

1. Short P–R interval (less than 0.12 s)
2. Widened QRS complex (greater than 0.12 s)
3. Delta wave: This is the slurred upstroke of QRS complex (Fig. 10.14b, c)
4. Secondary S–T segment, T wave change

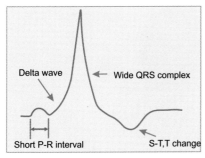

Delta wave   ← Wide QRS complex

Short P-R interval   S-T,T change

Fig. 10.14b   Wolf–Parkinson–White (WPW) syndrome. Note the delta wave, short P–R interval, wide QRS complex, and the accompanying S–T segment, T wave change.

Depending on the location of the accessory pathway in relation to the sino-atrial node and the relative transmission characteristics of the accessory pathway and the AV node, the morphology of ECG may vary from a classic presentation to near normal.

The treatment of pre-excitation mainly involves removal of the accessory pathway. The pathway is detected precisely by electrophysiological studies and then removed by radiofrequency catheter ablation (Fig. 10.14d).

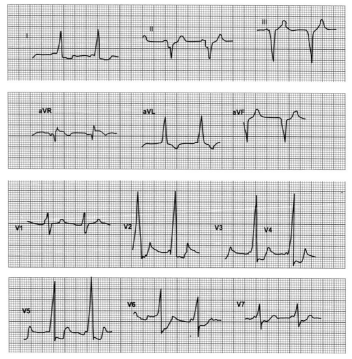

Fig. 10.14c   WPW syndrome. This ECG is taken from a 40-year-old man who presented with paroxysmal supraventricular tachycardia (PSVT). After termination of PSVT, the ECG revealed WPW syndrome. Note the wide QRS complexes with delta waves and short P–R interval.

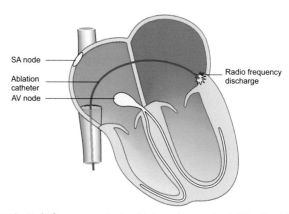

Fig. 10.14d   Radiofrequency catheter ablation of bypass tract. AV node, atrioventricular node; SA node, sino-atrial node.

PACEMAKER

A pacemaker (or artificial pacemaker) is a battery-powered medical device that uses electrical current, delivered by electrodes contacting the heart muscles, to regulate the beating of the heart. The primary purpose of a pacemaker is to maintain an adequate heart rate and rhythm, either because the heart's native pacemaker is not fast enough or there is a block in the heart's electrical conduction system.

Pacing is mainly of two types: temporary and permanent.

Temporary Pacing

In temporary transvenous pacing, the pacemaker electrode is placed under sterile conditions via a central venous catheter through transvenous route (internal juglar vein, subclavian vein, or femoral vein). The proximal tip of the electrode is placed into either the right atrium or right ventricle. The other end of the electrode is attached to the pulse generator, outside the body. The endocardium is stimulated directly by electric current that is supplied by the pulse generator. Batteries are kept in the generator housing.

Permanent Pacing

Permanent pacing is done in cardiac catheterization laboratory under intravenous conscious sedation and local anaesthesia. Permanent pacing with an implantable pacemaker involves placement of one or more pacing electrodes within the chambers of the heart, either right atrium or right ventricle or both in dual chamber pacing, via the cephalic vein or the subclavian vein (Fig. 10.15a). One end of each electrode is attached to the muscle of the heart and the other end is attached to the pulse generator. Pulse generators contain, among other things, a battery, an output circuit, a sensing circuit, and a timing circuit. The battery most commonly used in permanent pacers is a lithium–iodide type and has a life span of 5–8 years. Most commonly, the pulse generator is placed below the subcutaneous fat of the chest wall, above the muscles and bones of the chest either in right or left pectoral area.

The two most important features to identify the paced rhythm is the presence of pacemaker spikes and the broad QRS complex (Fig. 10.15b, c).

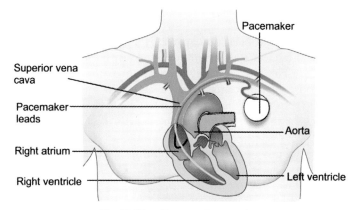

Fig. 10.15a   Permanent pacemaker.

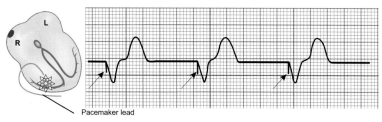

Fig. 10.15b   Illustration of pacemaker function. Note the pacing spikes (arrows) followed by broad QRS complex.

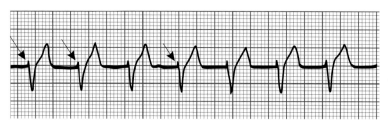

Fig. 10.15c   Normal pacemaker function. Note the pacing spikes (arrows) and the broad QRS complexes.

BIBLIOGRAPHY

1. Aquilina O. A brief history of cardiac pacing. *Images Paediatr Cardiol* 2006; 27, 17–81.
2. Arora R, Mukhopadhyay S, Yusuf J, et al. Technique, results, and follow-up of interventional treatment of rheumatic mitral stenosis in children. *Cardiol Young* 2007; 17(1), 3–11.

3. Bashour FA and Cochran PW. The association of electrical alternans with pericardial effusion. *Dis Chest* 1963; 44, 146–153.

4. Berman L and Schamroth L. Acute pulmonary embolism. *Heart and Lung* 1979; 8, 1146–1147.

5. Choi YS, Choi EK and Oh S. Typical atrioventricular nodal reentrant tachycardia in a patient with fasciculoventricular pathway. *J Electrocardiol* 2007; 40(6), 535–538.

6. Corey S and Richard J. ABC of clinical electrocardiography: conditions not primarily affecting the heart. *BMJ* 2002; 324, 1320–1323.

7. Durrer D, Schuilenburg RM and Wellens HJ. Pre-excitation revisited. *Am J Cardiol* 1970; 25(6), 690–697.

8. Ellenbogen KA. *Clinical Cardiac Pacing.* W.B. Saunders, 1995.

9. Furman S. A Practice of Cardiac Pacing. Futura Publishing, 1993.

10. Gaita F, Giustetto C, Riccardi R, et al. Wolff-Parkinson-White syndrome. Identification and management. *Drugs* 1992; 43(2), 185–200.

11. Giardina AC, Ehlers KH and Engle MA. Wolff-Parkinson-White syndrome in infants and children. A long-term follow-up study. *Br Heart J* 1972; 34(8), 839–846.

12. Ibars S, Anguera I, Gusi G, et al. Myocardial metastases presenting as ventricular tachycardia. *J Electrocardiol* 2007; 40(4), 365–367.

13. McGavigan AD, Clark E, Quinn FR, et al. Localization of accessory pathways in the Wolff-Parkinson-White pattern—physician versus computer interpretation of the same algorithm. *Pacing Clin Electrophysiol* 2007; 30(8), 998–1002.

14. Perosio AM, Suarez LD, Bunster AM, et al. Preexcitation syndrome and hypertrophic cardiomyopathy. *J Electrocardiol* 1983; 16, 29–40.

15. Robert WC and Day PJ. Electrocardiographic observations in clinically isolated, pure and chronic severe aortic regurgitation. Analysis of 30 necropsy patients aged 19 to 65 years. *Am J Cardiol* 1985; 55, 432–438.

16. Schamroth L. *An Introduction to Electrocardiography*, Seventh edition, Blackwell Science (Indian Reprint), 2002; pp. 189–309.

17. Scott RC. The electrocardiogram in ventricular septal defect. *Am Heart J* 1961; 62, 842-844.

18. Siegel RJ and Roberts WC. Electrocardiographic observations in severe aortic stenosis: correlative necropsy study of clinical, haemodynamic, and ECG variables demonstrating relation of 12-lead QRS amplitude to peak systolic transaortic pressure gradient. *Am Heart J* 1982; 103, 210-221.

19. Silver HM and Calatayud JB. Evaluation of QRS criteria in patients with chronic obstructive pulmonary disease. *Chest* 1971; 59, 153–159.

20. Sodi-Pallers D and Marsico F. The importance of electrocardiographic patterns in congenital heart disease. *Am Heart J* 1955; 49, 202-217.

21. Wall K, Oddsson H, Ternestedt BM, et al. Thirty-year electrocardiographic follow-up after repair of tetralogy of Fallot or atrial septal defect. *J Electrocardiol* 2007; 40(2), 214–217.

CHAPTER 11

Method of Interpretation of ECG

INTRODUCTION

The interpretation of electrocardiogram (ECG) starts with the history and clinical examination of the patient. This is often the most neglected step. ECG should always be interpreted in light of the clinical findings. This gives us the clue based on which it becomes easier to read ECG. This step is very important for the beginners, as it enhances the accuracy of interpretation of ECG. Clinical diagnosis and ECG are complimentary to each other. The study of an ECG should be systematic otherwise important findings will be missed and the diagnosis will become difficult. The following points should be considered while studying an ECG to arrive at a diagnosis:

RATE

The rate should be calculated to rule out bradycardia or tachycardia.

RHYTHM

The rhythm should be checked in the beginning. It is important to observe if the rhythm is regular or irregular. If regular, it should be checked whether the complexes are originating from sino-atrial node (sinus rhythm) or from any supraventricular or ventricular focus. If irregular, it is important to rule out sinus arrhythmia in the beginning, i.e., before considering any supraventricular or ventricular arrhythmia. The relation between P wave and the QRS complex should be noted. If there are abnormalities then they should be written down and correlated with the clinical findings. Rhythm should always be examined in lead II or V1 or in a rhythm strip.

P–R INTERVAL

The P–R interval should be checked in the leads where the P waves are seen very clearly (e.g., lead II). Prolongation of the P–R interval indicates first-degree heart block. Short P–R interval with delta wave indicates Wolf–Parkinson–White syndrome.

P WAVES

It is important to rule out any right or left atrial enlargement by examination of P waves in all the 12 leads but especially in leads

II and V1. The P wave is always inverted in lead aVR and it may be biphasic in lead V1. If the P wave is upright in lead aVR, then there may be dextrocardia. Inverted P waves in leads II, III, and aVF indicate nodal/junctional rhythm.

QRS COMPLEXES

The QRS complexes should be studied in all the 12 leads and should be checked whether they are of normal configuration and correspond to the normal complexes in all the 12 leads. The following points should be studied in the QRS complexes:

1. Duration
2. Ventricular activation time (VAT)
3. Presence of normal or pathological Q waves
4. Amplitude of R and S waves
5. QRS axis: To rule out left or right axis deviation

T WAVES

It should be checked whether the T waves are upright or inverted. The T wave is normally inverted in lead aVR. Deep and symmetric T wave inversion is a sign of myocardial ischaemia. Asymmetric inversion is a feature of strain pattern associated with left or right ventricular hypertrophy (LVH or RVH).

U WAVES

It should be checked whether the U waves are present or absent. If present, they may be normal or may be a feature of hypokalaemia.

S–T SEGMENT

The S–T segment should be carefully examined to rule out any elevation or depression. An elevation in the segment indicates myocardial infarction or pericarditis or ventricular aneurysm while a depression indicates myocardial ischaemia. S–T segment depression with a reverse check sign or scooped S–T segment depression is a feature of digitalis effect.

LVH OR RVH

The presence of LVH or RVH should be checked. For LVH, one must look for the sum of amplitude of S wave in lead V1 and the amplitude of R wave in lead V5 or V6. If it is more than 35 mm, then one should look for rest of the features as described earlier. For RVH, one should look for the R:S ratio in lead V1. If it is more than 1, then one must look for the other features of RVH as described earlier.

CONDUCTION DISTURBANCE

Conduction disturbances such as first-, second-, and third-degree heart block should be checked. Left or right bundle branch block (LBBB or RBBB) should be excluded. If rSR' pattern is seen in lead V1, then look for other features of RBBB and if rSR' pattern is seen in lead V6, then look for other features of LBBB.

REPORTING OF ECG

ECG reporting should be done in details and the diagnosis should be mentioned clearly. ECG should be reported in the following format.

Name:_____ Age:_____ Sex:_____ Drugs:_____

Date & Time: _____

Rate: _____Rhythm: _____P wave: _____P–R interval: _____

Q–T interval: _____

QRS complex:

    (a)   Configuration_____
    (b)   Duration_____
    (c)   QRS axis_____
    (d)   VAT_____
          S–T segment:_____

T wave: _____
U wave: _____
Diagnosis: _____

GLOSSARY

This section is intended as a review for students and beginners. In this section, some of the important questions students often face in their examination and the practical problems beginners often face at the bedside are mentioned. However, the theoretical details are not discussed here and the reader should consult the text for details.

1. Always treat the patient and not the electrocardiogram (ECG).
2. Before analyzing the results of ECG, ensure that all the 12 leads are recorded and there is proper standardization.
3. In lead aVR, all the complexes are **negative.**
4. The P–R interval is 0.12–0.20 s. It is prolonged in 1° heart block and shortened in Wolf–Parkinson–White (WPW) syndrome.
5. Normal Q–T interval is 0.35–0.42 s. The most important cause of Q–T interval prolongation is **hypocalcaemia.**
6. A normal q wave is seen in leads I, II, aVF, and V4–V6.
7. R wave is the dominant wave in leads V4–V6 and S wave is the dominant wave in leads V1 and V2.
8. U wave is in the same direction as that of the T wave. Prominent U wave is seen in **hypokalaemia.**
9. T wave may be normally inverted in leads V1–V3. Tall and peaked T wave is seen in **hyperkalaemia.**
10. In early repolarization syndrome, the S–T segment is elevated. This is often confused with **myocardial infarction.** Early repolarization syndrome is a normal variant of ECG.
11. The normal QRS axis is **–30° to +90°.** While analyzing an ECG it is not always important to calculate the exact axis but detection of a change in axis is more important.
12. **Rule of thumb for axis determination:** If the dominant deflections in leads I and aVF are positive, then the axis is normal. If there is positive deflection in lead I and negative deflection in lead aVF, then there is left axis deviation. If there is negative deflection in lead I and positive deflection in lead aVF, then there is right axis deviation.

13. To detect left ventricular hypertrophy (LVH), first calculate SV1 + RV5 or RV6 which is **more than 35 mm in LVH.** Then look for other abnormalities such as S–T segment, T wave change, left axis deviation, and increase in ventricular activation time (VAT) in leads V5 and V6.

14. To detect right ventricular hypertrophy (RVH), first calculate the R:S ratio in lead VI, which is **more than 1 in RVH.** Then look for other features such as S–T segment, T wave change, and increase in VAT in lead V1.

15. To detect bundle branch block look for rSR' pattern; if it is present in lead V1, then there is right bundle branch block and if it is present in lead V6, then there is left bundle branch block. Along with it look for the widening of QRS complex (more than 0.12 s), S–T segment, T wave change.

16. To detect left-anterior hemiblock (LAHB), calculate the QRS axis (left axis deviation) and then look for the depth of S waves in leads II and III. In LAHB, the depth of S wave in lead III is more than that in lead II.

17. If there is rapid ventricular (narrow QRS) rate, then look for P waves. If present, then consider sinus tachycardia. If the P waves are not seen and R–R interval is regular, then consider paroxysmal atrial tachycardia, but if the interval is irregular, consider atrial fibrillation.

18. If there is broad QRS complex with a very slow ventricular rate with atrioventricular dissociation, then consider **complete heart block.**

19. Concave upwards S–T segment elevation is seen in acute pericarditis and early repolarization syndrome.

20. Convex upwards S–T segment elevation is seen in acute myocardial infarction and ventricular aneurysm.

21. Deep Q wave is the **surest sign of old myocardial infarction.** The duration of pathological Q wave is more than 0.04 s and the Q wave is more than 25% of the R wave amplitude.

22. Presence of complete pause after extrasystole indicates ventricular origin and incomplete pause indicates atrial origin.

23. Inverted P wave in leads II, III, and aVF indicates **nodal or junctional rhythm.**

24. In accelerated idioventricular rhythm, the ventricular rate is **slow** (60–100 beats/min).

25. In Torsades de pointes there is twisting of points. It is associated with **prolongation of Q–T interval.**
26. **Delta wave** is seen in WPW syndrome. The P–R interval is short in this syndrome.
27. **P mitrale** indicates left atrial hypertrophy.
28. **P pulmonale** indicates right atrial hypertrophy.
29. **Dextrocardia** is diagnosed by interchanging complexes in leads aVR and aVL.
30. T inversion in leads V1–V3 indicates **persistent juvenile pattern.**
31. **Mirror image of check sign** is seen in digitalis effect.
32. **J waves or Osborne waves** are seen in hypothermia.
33. **SI, QIII, and TIII** is seen in acute pulmonary embolism.
34. **Electrical alternans** is seen in pericardial effusion.
35. **rsR' complex** in lead V1 with right axis deviation is seen in **ostium secundum** type of atrial septal defect.
36. **rsR' complex** in lead V1 with left axis deviation is seen in **ostium primum** type of atrial septal defect.
37. Gradual prolongation of P–R interval followed by a dropped beat indicates **Wenckebach phenomenon.**
38. **Fibrillatory wave** is seen in atrial fibrillation.
39. **Saw tooth wave** is seen in atrial flutter.
40. **Concordance pattern** is seen in ventricular tachycardia.

INDEX